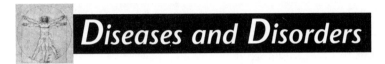

Diseases and Disorders

Smallpox

Titles in the Diseases and Disorders series include:

Alzheimer's Disease
Anorexia and Bulimia
Arthritis
Asthma
Attention Deficit Disorder
Autism
Breast Cancer
Cerebral Palsy
Chronic Fatigue Syndrome
Cystic Fibrosis
Down Syndrome
Diabetes
Epilepsy
Hemophilia
Hepatitis
Learning Disabilities
Leukemia
Lyme Disease
Multiple Sclerosis
Phobias
Schizophrenia
Sexually Transmitted Diseases
Sleep Disorders
West Nile Virus

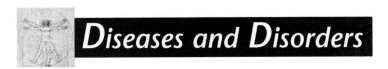
Diseases and Disorders

Smallpox

Barbara Saffer

LUCENT BOOKS®

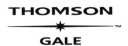
THOMSON
™
GALE

San Diego • Detroit • New York • San Francisco • Cleveland
New Haven, Conn. • Waterville, Maine • London • Munich

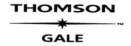

On cover: A doctor administers the smallpox
vaccine to schoolchildren in this 1947 photo.

LIBRARY OF CONGRESS CATALOGING-IN-PUBLICATION DATA

Saffer, Barbara.
   Smallpox / by Barbara Saffer.
      p. cm. — (Diseases and disorders)
Includes bibliographical references and index.
Summary: Provides a historical overview of the dreaded disease, including its centuries-
long effects on society, its causes and symptoms, the development of a vaccine, the
eradication of the disease, and its present-day potential as a weapon of war.
   ISBN 1-59018-301-0 (hbk. : alk. paper)
   1. Smallpox—Juvenile literature. I. Title. II. Diseases and disorders series
   RC183 .S26 2003
   616.9'12—dc21
                                                                      2002154020

Printed in the United States of America

Table of Contents

Foreword   6

Introduction
    A Disease "Most Fearful to Behold"   8

Chapter 1
    What Is Smallpox?   11

Chapter 2
    The Scourge and Its History   22

Chapter 3
    Inoculation to Prevent Epidemics   35

Chapter 4
    The Smallpox Vaccine Is Developed   48

Chapter 5
    Smallpox Is Eradicated   64

Chapter 6
    Smallpox as a Biological Weapon   75

    Notes   89
    Glossary   94
    Organizations to Contact   96
    For Further Reading   97
    Works Consulted   98
    Index   104
    Picture Credits   111
    About the Author   112

"The Most Difficult Puzzles Ever Devised"

C HARLES BEST, ONE of the pioneers in the search for a cure for diabetes, once explained what it is about medical research that intrigued him so. "It's not just the gratification of knowing one is helping people," he confided, "although that probably is a more heroic and selfless motivation. Those feelings may enter in, but truly, what I find best is the feeling of going toe to toe with nature, of trying to solve the most difficult puzzles ever devised. The answers are there somewhere, those keys that will solve the puzzle and make the patient well. But how will those keys be found?"

Since the dawn of civilization, nothing has so puzzled people— and often frightened them, as well—as the onset of illness in a body or mind that had seemed healthy before. A seizure, the inability of a heart to pump, the sudden deterioration of muscle tone in a small child—being unable to reverse such conditions or even to understand why they occur was unspeakably frustrating to healers. Even before there were names for such conditions, even before they were understood at all, each was a reminder of how complex the human body was, and how vulnerable.

While our grappling with understanding diseases has been frustrating at times, it has also provided some of humankind's most heroic accomplishments. Alexander Fleming's accidental discovery in 1928 of a mold that could be turned into penicillin

6

has resulted in the saving of untold millions of lives. The isolation of the enzyme insulin has reversed what was once a death sentence for anyone with diabetes. There have been great strides in combating conditions for which there is not yet a cure, too. Medicines can help AIDS patients live longer, diagnostic tools such as mammography and ultrasounds can help doctors find tumors while they are treatable, and laser surgery techniques have made the most intricate, minute operations routine.

This "toe-to-toe" competition with diseases and disorders is even more remarkable when seen in a historical continuum. An astonishing amount of progress has been made in a very short time. Just two hundred years ago, the existence of germs as a cause of some diseases was unknown. In fact, it was less than 150 years ago that a British surgeon named Joseph Lister had difficulty persuading his fellow doctors that washing their hands before delivering a baby might increase the chances of a healthy delivery (especially if they had just attended to a diseased patient)!

Each book in Lucent's *Diseases and Disorders* series explores a disease or disorder and the knowledge that has been accumulated (or discarded) by doctors through the years. Each book also examines the tools used for pinpointing a diagnosis, as well as the various means that are used to treat or cure a disease. Finally, new ideas are presented—techniques or medicines that may be on the horizon.

Frustration and disappointment are still part of medicine, for not every disease or condition can be cured or prevented. But the limitations of knowledge are being pushed outward constantly; the "most difficult puzzles ever devised" are finding challengers every day.

A Disease "Most Fearful to Behold"

F OR THOUSANDS OF years, smallpox was one of the world's most dreaded scourges. Caused by the Variola virus, this highly contagious disease is characterized by an extensive burning rash that erupts into pus-filled pocks, or pustules, that smell like rotting flesh. In 1634, the Puritan leader William Bradford wrote of Native Americans suffering from smallpox: "They lie on hard mats, the pox breaking and mattering [oozing pus], and running one into another, their skin cleaving [sticking] . . . to the mats they lie on; when they turn them, a whole side will flea [peel] off at once . . . and they will be all of a gore blood, most fearful to behold."[1] Many smallpox victims died horribly, while survivors were scarred, and sometimes blinded, for life. An early account from Brazil described "pox that were so rotten and poisonous that the flesh fell off,"[2] and Gregory of Tours depicted the body of a nobleman who died of smallpox in A.D. 580 as "black and burnt, as if it had laid on a coal fire."[3]

The affliction caused by Variola was named "the small pockes" (smallpox) in the early sixteenth century to distinguish its spots from the larger ones caused by syphilis, an infectious bacterial disease. The rash caused by syphilis was called "the great pockes." By the twentieth century, hundreds of millions of people had died as a result of smallpox.

In the late 1790s, Edward Jenner developed a smallpox vaccine, and in 1958 the World Health Organization (WHO) began a campaign to eradicate the disease. After a grueling worldwide crusade, the WHO finally announced in 1979 that smallpox had been eliminated from the earth. The last victim of naturally occurring small-

8

pox was Ali Maow Maalin, a twenty-three-year-old cook in Somalia. When Maalin recovered in November 1977, health officials thought smallpox had been conquered. They were shocked, therefore, when Janet Parker—a medical photographer in Birmingham, England—contracted smallpox ten months later.

Parker was the victim of a bizarre medical accident. Her photography studio at the University of Birmingham was in the same building as a viral research laboratory run by Professor Henry Bedson. The Variola virus that Bedson had been researching had escaped from his laboratory, entered a service duct, and drifted to a room that Parker used. Janet Parker died from smallpox on September 11, 1978, the last known person to perish from the disease. Professor Bedson, racked with guilt and anguished by public blame, committed suicide.

After smallpox was eradicated, all samples of the Variola virus were supposed to be sent to two laboratories, one in the United States and one in the former Soviet Union. Scientists there planned

Somalia native Ali Maow Maalin suffered from the world's last recorded case of endemic smallpox in October 1977.

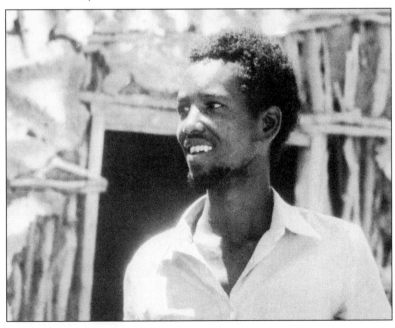

to study the viruses and then destroy them. The destruction date has been repeatedly postponed, however, out of fear that "secret" Variola samples were kept by some countries and might fall into the hands of terrorists.

Fear of bioterrorism intensified in the fall of 2001, after victims in Florida, New Jersey, New York, and Washington, D.C., became infected with anthrax that had been dispersed though the mail. Health officials worry that other biological weapons could spread plague, botulism, tularemia, hemorrhagic fever, Lassa fever, or smallpox. To prevent the disaster that could be unleashed by a smallpox epidemic, researchers want to continue studying Variola so that they can develop better vaccines and medicines.

Chapter 1

What Is Smallpox?

S MALLPOX IS A severe, contagious viral disease. The scientific name for the virus that causes smallpox, Variola, comes from the Latin word *varius,* which means "spotted." Variola has no animal carrier; it infects only humans. It is transmitted from person to person through the air. Variola spreads when smallpox sufferers talk, cough, or sneeze, or when they leak pus from ruptured pocks onto clothes, bedding, and other items. Such contaminated objects can remain infectious for months and carry Variola over long distances. In the 1880s, for example, a smallpox outbreak in Pecos, Texas, was traced to a silk handkerchief lying along the railroad track, which was thought to have been thrown from a passenger train. Victims' corpses can also spread Variola to people who prepare the corpses for burial.

Variola viruses enter people when they inhale, coming in through the nose and mouth. The incubation period, which lasts from one to three weeks, follows. During this time, the victim feels normal. After the incubation period, the victim begins to feel ill. Most deaths occur about two weeks after the first signs of illness. In rare cases, however, death occurs almost immediately. A European settler writing about North American Indians in the nineteenth century observed, "[Smallpox] kills a greater part of them before any eruption [rash] appears."[4]

The Variola Virus

Viruses are tiny, simple organisms composed of a strand of genetic material surrounded by a protein coat. A virus's genetic material, either DNA (deoxyribonucleic acid) or RNA (ribonucleic acid), is divided into genes, which pass on the organism's traits from one generation to the next. Viruses *must* enter the cells of other living things to reproduce, and each kind of virus attacks one or more specific host organisms.

All poxviruses belong to a group called orthopoxviruses, which have similar structures and genetic material. Poxviruses are larger than most viruses. They include the human smallpox virus, variola, as well as leporipoxviruses, which attack rabbits and hares; avipoxviruses, which attack birds; capripoxviruses, which attack sheep and goats; and monkeypox viruses, which attack monkeys and squirrels. Other poxviruses cause cowpox, sealpox, deerpox, skunkpox, peacockpox, kangaroopox, buffalopox, camelpox, gerbilpox, and so on.

A young girl with an orthopoxvirus exhibits monkeypox lesions on her hand and leg.

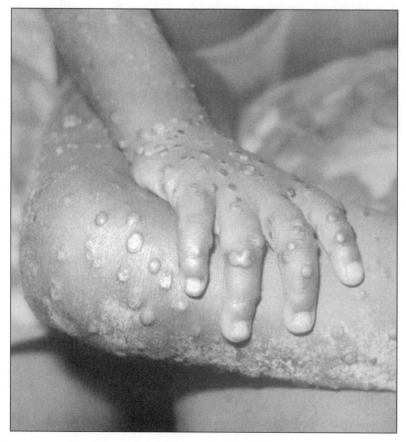

Replication Cycle of Smallpox

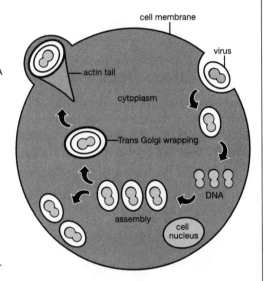

Clockwise from top right:

A smallpox virus enters the host cell. It releases its DNA and begins to make copies of itself. The new viruses are assembled. Most (bottom left) remain inside the host cell and will be released when the cell bursts. Others receive a second wrapping of host cell membrane at the Trans Golgi. Actin tails help them push their way to the cell surface, where they will be released to infect new cells.

cell membrane

virus

actin tail

cytoplasm

Trans Golgi wrapping

DNA

assembly

cell nucleus

Variola is among the most complex of human viruses. Each smallpox virus has about two hundred genes in its DNA strand; by comparison, the polio virus, yellow fever virus, and measles virus have fewer than ten genes each. Variola viruses look like tiny hand grenades. They are oval-shaped particles about four hundred nanometers long and two hundred nanometers wide (one nanometer is equal to one-millionth of a millimeter), with ridged surfaces covered with spikes.

To enter a human cell, Variola connects to receptors on the cell surface. It then slips through the cell membrane and enters the cytoplasm, the liquid material inside the cell. As soon as Variola penetrates the cell, it takes over the cell's reproductive machinery and sets up something akin to a viral factory. The factory produces large quantities of viral enzymes, viral DNA, viral proteins, and so on. These viral components are assembled into hundreds of thousands of new Variola viruses, which emerge from the cell. The liberated viruses spread to neighboring cells, to other parts of the body, or to other people.

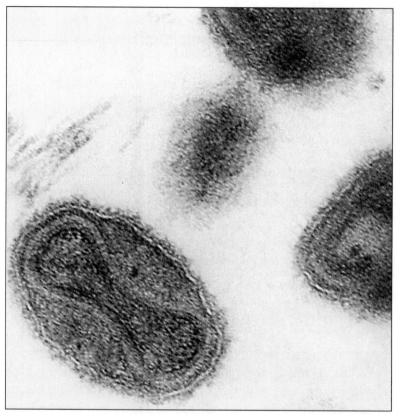

An oval-shaped Variola major virus particle (pictured) is seen under a microscope. This strain of the Variola virus produces the more lethal forms of smallpox.

Variola Major and Variola Minor

There are at least two strains of the Variola virus that cause smallpox: Variola major and Variola minor. Variola major is the more virulent, or lethal, strain. It causes a severe illness, with a typical death rate of about 30 percent. Variola major is responsible for the two most dangerous types of smallpox, hemorrhagic smallpox and malignant smallpox. These rare forms of the disease are even more deadly than common smallpox. Hemorrhagic smallpox is marked by heavy bleeding in the skin and internal organs and is always fatal. Malignant smallpox is characterized by connecting, dark, velvety flat pocks. Few people survive this form of the illness, and those that do often lose large patches of skin.

The less virulent strain, Variola minor, causes a milder illness, with a death rate of about 1 percent. "Mild smallpox" is usually called alastrim but is also known by many other names, including cottonpox, whitepox, Cuban itch, Manila scab, and West Indian smallpox. People with alastrim develop an extensive rash, like that of Variola major, but it leaves few scars.

The Disease

Smallpox viruses are sensitive to heat and humidity, so the disease spreads most easily in winter and early spring. Smallpox victims become infectious, or capable of transmitting the disease, shortly before the rash appears. The initial rash, which consists of red spots in the nose and throat, erupts after an incubation period of seven to twenty-one days. The red spots shed Variola viruses into the saliva. Thus, when the sick person speaks, coughs, or sneezes, viruses are sprayed into the air—where other people can breathe them in. Medical journalist Richard Preston notes, "If you inhale a single particle of smallpox, you can come down with the disease."[5]

When people inhale air contaminated with smallpox, Variola enters through the mouth and nose. In *susceptible* individuals, the viruses then infect the respiratory system and local lymph nodes and multiply. After a few days, millions of viruses enter the blood-stream, travel to internal organs (such as the liver, spleen, lungs, bone marrow, and additional lymph nodes), and undergo *another* multiplication cycle. A week or two later, viruses enter the blood-stream once again and travel to the skin. At this stage, when huge numbers of viruses are circulating, the victim exhibits the first symptoms of the disease. These symptoms may include fever, headache, backache, fatigue, weakness, abdominal pain, vomiting, pain in the arms and legs, and delirium (mental disturbances). The symptoms usually appear suddenly and last two to six days. When these symptoms subside, the rash begins to erupt.

When the fever diminishes, the rash appears, starting out as small red dots on the mouth, tongue, palate, and pharynx. Over the next day or two, skin lesions, or spots, appear. Initially, flat red spots, called macules, break out on the face and upper limbs. The spots then spread to the trunk, lower limbs, palms, and soles. The macules, filled with Variola viruses, are most dense on the face, arms, and legs.

Over the next two weeks or so, the rash progresses from macules to pustules. First, the macules form elevated spots called papules. The papules fill with fluid and become vesicles. The vesicles, in turn, become engorged with pus, to form pustules. Describing a smallpox victim, Preston wrote, "The [pustules] were hard and dry, and they didn't leak. They were like ball bearings, embedded in the skin."[6] At the height of the illness, many patients feel as if their skin is on fire, their bodies appear scalded or burned, and they develop a revolting odor, like rotting flesh. Smallpox deaths, when they occur, usually happen during this phase. According to Preston, "Death comes with a breathing arrest or a heart attack or shock or an immune-system storm, though exactly how smallpox kills a person is not known."[7] Physicians suggest that death may result from the toxemia, or blood poisoning, caused by large amounts of immune system chemicals associated with Variola viruses.

If the patient survives the pustule phase, the pocks dry up, scabs form, and the patient begins to recover. The scabs fall off in ten days to two weeks, leaving survivors with deep, pitted scars. These light-colored scars, or pockmarks, are especially dense on the face. In most cases, the disease, from initial infection to the loss of all scabs, lasts from four to six weeks. Smallpox patients are contagious from just before the rash appears until the scabs drop off, but the dried scabs themselves can remain infectious for years.

Complications

Smallpox victims sometimes experience complications, or secondary effects, from the disease. A common problem is secondary bacterial infection of the lesions. If massive numbers of bacteria migrate from the lesions to the bloodstream, septicemia, or blood poisoning, may result, causing chills, fever, weakness, and infection of internal organs.

Other complications involve inflammation of various organs. Inflammation of a body part causes tissue damage, pain, heat, red-

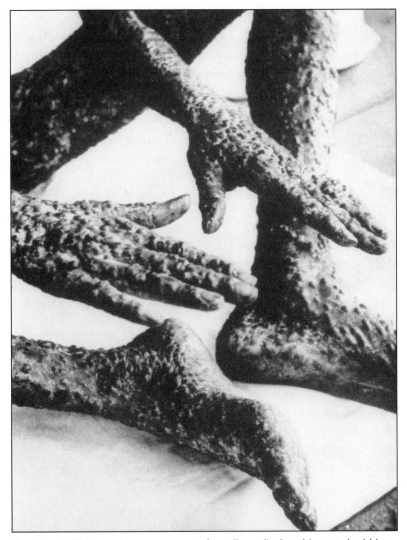

A patient afflicted with a severe case of smallpox displays his pustule-ridden hands and feet.

ness, swelling, and an inability to function properly. Respiratory complications, which are common, include inflammation of the bronchial tubes (bronchitis) or lungs (pneumonia), which may be fatal. Inflammation of the brain (encephalitis), most common in adults, can lead to fever, headache, double vision, deafness, hallucinations, delusions, and coma. This may also be fatal.

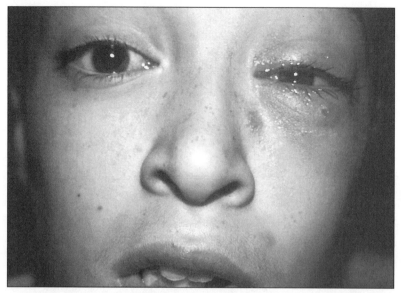

A twelve-year-old boy with smallpox suffers from keratitis, or inflammation of the cornea.

Smallpox pustules near or on the eyes can lead to inflammation of the cornea (keratitis), inner eyelids (conjunctivitis), or iris (iritis), as well as cause damage to the optic nerve. If the injury is severe, blindness results. In children, inflammation of the joints (arthritis) and bones (osteomyelitis) sometimes occurs. This can lead to growth problems, swollen joints, malformed bones, stubby fingers, and fused joints that are incapable of bending. Finally, if a pregnant woman contracts smallpox, the disease may infect, and sometimes kill, the fetus.

Diagnosis

Doctors diagnose, or identify, a disease by examining its symptoms. To diagnose smallpox, physicians must differentiate it from other rash-causing diseases. Historically, smallpox was often confused with measles, a contagious disease marked by fever, sneezing, a runny nose, and small red spots on the skin. For the first few days, the smallpox rash resembles the measles rash. Measles spots, however, begin to disappear after two or three days; smallpox spots, on the other hand, grow larger and become pustules.

Smallpox also looks similar to chicken pox, an infectious illness characterized by fever, sore throat, cough, weakness, and lesions that change from papules, to vesicles, to pustules. However, on any part of the body, such as the face, trunk, or limbs, the lesions of smallpox are the same age, or at the same stage of development, and look alike; chicken pox lesions, on the other hand, vary in age and appearance. Chicken pox spots are also most dense on the torso, whereas smallpox spots are most concentrated on the face and limbs. Moreover, smallpox spots spread to the palms of the hands and the soles of the feet, while chicken pox spots do not. Finally, smallpox lesions extend deeper into the skin, and cause more damage, than chicken pox spots.

Smallpox victims also have a distinctive smell. Preston described the odor of a smallpox victim: "[It was] a sweet, sickly, cloying odor. . . . It was not the smell of decay, for his skin was

Spots caused by chicken pox (pictured) are usually concentrated on the patient's torso, while smallpox lesions more commonly appear on the face and limbs.

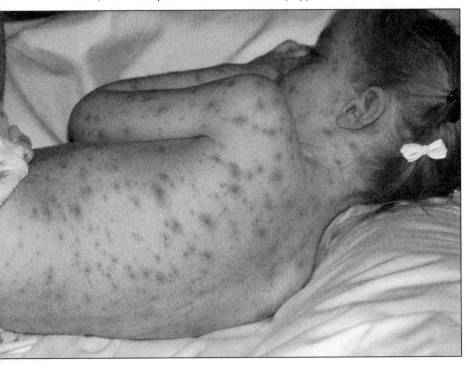

sealed. The pus within the skin was throwing off gases that diffused out of his body."[8] During epidemics, the odor of a house or hospital ward containing smallpox patients could be particularly repellent. According to Dr. Nicholas Ward, who worked in Africa, "I've spent a fair amount of my life working with tropical diseases, and I can truly say there is nothing so awful as a case of smallpox, particularly the type where a person becomes a bloody mess. . . . I would have a shrewd idea of a diagnosis after walking into a home. I could smell it."[9]

If a person is suspected to have smallpox, the diagnosis can be confirmed by growing Variola viruses from skin lesions or observing the viruses with an electron microscope. The specific strain of virus, Variola major or Variola minor, can be identified by taking blood samples from the smallpox victim and testing the viral DNA with specific enzymes.

Treatment and Recovery

Although scientists have learned a great deal about smallpox, they have not yet developed a cure for the disease. Treatment generally consists of isolating patients and making them comfortable. If secondary bacterial infections occur, antibiotics (substances that kill bacteria) are prescribed.

Meanwhile, the victim's body mounts a furious offense against the disease. Six days after the rash appears (about twenty-one days after infection), the patient's immune system starts to produce large amounts of antibodies, immune system cells, and chemicals to kill the viruses. If the immune response is strong enough, the Variola viruses are destroyed, and the patient recovers. If the immune response is too weak, the victim dies. Researchers suggest that the worst cases of smallpox—hemorrhagic smallpox and malignant smallpox—may result from defective immune systems.

Although there are no known medicines that can cure smallpox once its symptoms are present, scientists continue to search for antiviral treatments. Research shows that cidofovir, a drug that interferes with DNA replication, may help prevent smallpox if given within a day or two after a person has been exposed to the Variola virus. Experiments have also indicated that more than twenty-five other substances, including new classes of drugs, may work against Variola.

Because officials have become concerned about a possible biological attack with smallpox, the Centers for Disease Control (CDC) in Atlanta has dedicated one of its two maximum-containment laboratories (those that are most secure) to smallpox-only research. There, scientists are working furiously to learn more about Variola, its control, and its origins.

Chapter 2

The Scourge and Its History

N O ONE KNOWS where or when smallpox viruses first attacked humans. Many scientists think that Variola started out as an animal virus—perhaps of rodents or cattle—that slowly adapted to people. This is happening today with monkeypox, a disease similar to smallpox, which is spreading among people in central Africa.

Variola probably transferred to humans thousands of years ago. Archaeologists speculate that smallpox first became widespread among humans in ancient Egypt at least thirty-five hundred years ago, striking commoners and royalty alike. The mummy of the Egyptian pharaoh Ramses V, who died in 1157 B.C., has smallpox scars on the well-preserved skin of the face, neck, and arms.

After smallpox became endemic (firmly established) in ancient Egypt, it slowly spread around the world. Early epidemics thought to be caused by smallpox struck people in Turkey in 1346 B.C.; Athens, Greece, in 430 B.C.; Syracuse, Sicily, in 395 B.C.; Mecca, Saudi Arabia, in A.D. 570; Korea in 583; and Japan in 585. Smallpox also migrated along trade routes to China, Persia (modern-day Iran), and India. An Indian medical book written in A.D. 400 describes a disease that is probably smallpox: "The pustules are red, yellow, and white and they are accompanied with burning pain. . . . The skin seems studded with grains of rice." [10] In an attempt to protect themselves from the curse of smallpox, many cultures worshiped a smallpox god or goddess.

Turning to Religion

To guard themselves against the disease, people in India worshiped a smallpox goddess named Sitala, which means "the cool one."

Historians think the name comes from Sitala's supposed ability to relieve the high fever and burning sensation of smallpox. At temples devoted to Sitala, worshipers prayed that the goddess would either prevent smallpox or provide a cure.

In China, people revered a smallpox goddess called T'ou-Shen Niang-Niang. When smallpox struck, a drawing of the goddess was placed in the victim's home, and offerings were made to it. If

An effigy of the Indian goddess of smallpox, Sitala. Devout Hindus prayed regularly to Sitala to provide protection from the disease.

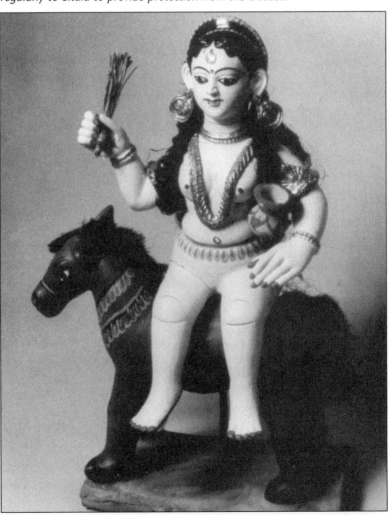

the victim recovered, the picture was carried from the home and ceremonially burned. If the patient died, the picture was torn up, and the goddess's spirit was chased from the home with curses.

The Japanese displayed a picture of Chinzei Hachiro Tametomo, a heroic Japanese archer, to ward off or cure smallpox. According

A nineteenth-century Japanese illustration depicts Chinzei Hachiro Tametomo driving away smallpox demons. The legendary archer was implored to spare the islands from infection.

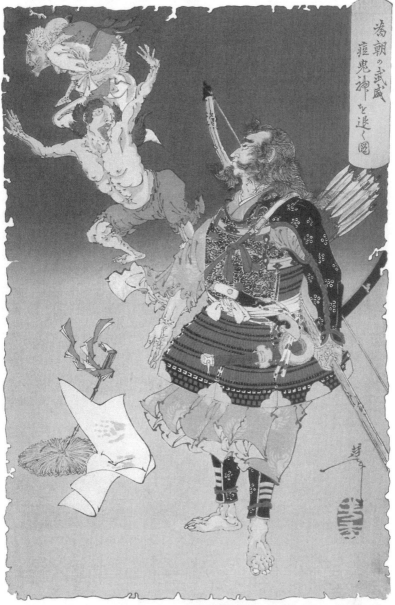

to legend, Tametomo prevented the smallpox demon from landing on the island of Oshimoa in the twelfth century, protecting the island's people from the disease.

Between about 400 B.C. and A.D. 1400, smallpox spread throughout Europe and Africa. In Europe, people prayed to Saint Nicaise, a fifth-century bishop of Reims, France, to protect them from smallpox. According to legend, Nicaise cured himself of smallpox with holy oil. A year later, when the Asian Huns, led by the ferocious warrior Attila, invaded Reims, Nicaise marched forth singing hymns. A Hun soldier chopped off the top of Nicaise's head, but the bishop continued to sing before he died. Afterward, smallpox forced the Huns to retreat. As a result, Nicaise became the French patron saint of smallpox.

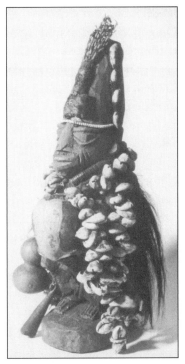

Shapona is a smallpox god worshiped by the Yoruba people of West Africa.

Smallpox gods in Africa were variously called Obaluaye, Omolu, Sagbata, and Shapona. The Yoruba people of West Africa believed that Shapona controlled the earth. "It was thought that the god of the earth, who nourished man by giving him maize [corn] . . . and all other grains of the earth, when moved to punishment caused the grains men had eaten to come out on their skins [as smallpox]." [11]

Folk Treatments

Until the middle of the nineteenth century, no one knew what caused smallpox. Various cultures blamed the disease on angry gods, deadly gases, and imbalances in body fluids. Thus, some folk treatments involved bleeding smallpox patients until they fainted, then exposing them to intense heat. Other popular therapies included palm oil, laxatives, fat from a donkey, vegetarianism, meditation, and dried horse dung. Charles Banister of Portland, Oregon, claimed that his family used dung tea as a remedy for generations: "The most . . . medicinal dung [was that] of the swine, the common sty-pig, which, when dried and baked in an oven and made into a tea is said to cure evils of all sorts, from the slightest indisposition to measles and smallpox." [12] Another popular treatment involved surrounding smallpox patients with the color red, which was thought to stimulate the blood and bring the infection to the surface. Thus, some smallpox victims were dressed in red clothes, wrapped in red blankets, placed under red lanterns, and had their rooms draped with red curtains.

Superstitions about smallpox were also common. Europeans tried to protect themselves from smallpox by covering their noses with vinegar-soaked rags, wearing charms made of animal teeth, hanging bags of camphor (now used to make mothballs) around their necks, and carrying tarred rope. A better way to control smallpox epidemics was quarantine, or isolation of smallpox patients. In eighteenth-century Europe and America, for example, smallpox patients were sometimes confined to ships in harbors or "pesthouses" on shore until they recovered or died.

Until smallpox was eradicated, frightful epidemics periodically plagued humankind. These became more frequent as large populations clustered in big cities. Moreover, when people began traveling from place to place—to discover riches, trade goods, spread religion, wage war, and so on—they took the smallpox virus with them. Thus, the disease eventually spread around the world.

Smallpox Spreads to Natives of the New World

In Old World cities, where smallpox was always lurking, about one-third of those who fell ill died from the disease. Survivors became immune, or resistant, to smallpox. Thus, after each epidemic, there was a lull, during which new babies were born and the susceptible population increased once more. When there were enough susceptible individuals, another smallpox epidemic would strike.

The death toll from smallpox was much higher among "virgin populations" that had not been previously exposed to the disease, like natives of the New World. Hence, when European explorers carried the deadly smallpox virus to Hispaniola, Mexico, Central America, and South America, the results were devastating. According to some historians, the native population of the New World, close to 72 million when Christopher Columbus landed in 1492, was reduced by war and disease to about six hundred thousand in 1800, one of the greatest losses in history.

Spanish Conquerors Disperse Smallpox to Hispaniola, Mexico, and South America

Smallpox first arrived in the New World with Columbus in 1492. The Spanish vessels that carried Columbus to Hispaniola (now Haiti and the Dominican Republic) also brought slaves with smallpox. By 1518, smallpox and other diseases, combined with Spanish

Explorers like Christopher Columbus brought smallpox from the Old World to the Americas, where the virus decimated native populations.

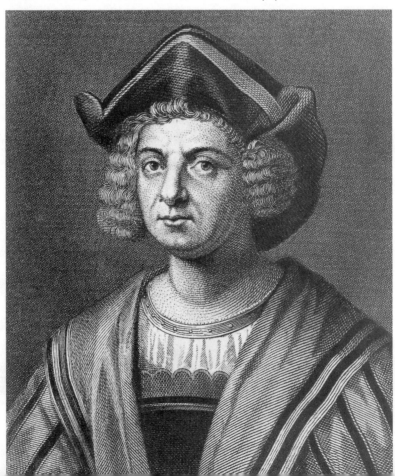

enslavement and cruelty, had reduced the native population there from nearly 8 million to twenty-three thousand. By 1535, almost all the natives of Hispaniola had been exterminated. Similar events occurred in Cuba and Puerto Rico. Moreover, when smallpox arrived on the American mainland, millions of natives—including the mighty empires of the Aztec and Inca—experienced some of the worst epidemic disasters of all time.

In 1519, the Spanish soldier and explorer Hernando Cortés, lured by tales of gold and riches, arrived in Mexico with five hundred fifty soldiers. The invaders made their way to Tenochtitlán (now Mexico City), where the Aztec emperor Montezuma—believing the Spaniards were descendants of the Aztec god Quetzalcoatl—

Aztec emperor Montezuma receives Spanish explorer Hernando Cortés in 1519. Cortés and his soldiers unknowingly carried smallpox into Mexico, killing 3 million Indians.

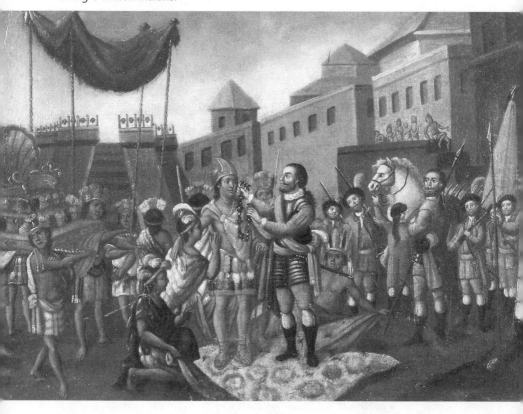

received them graciously. Cortés captured Montezuma and tried to rule the Aztec Empire through him. Soon after, in 1520, the Spanish officer Pánfilo de Narváez arrived in Mexico with nine hundred men to capture and replace Cortés. Cortés and a band of soldiers hurried off to confront Narváez and quickly defeated him. During the struggle, one of Cortés's men contracted smallpox from a slave on Narváez's ship.

While Cortés was away, the Aztec rebelled. They ousted the Spanish soldiers left behind and chased off Cortés when he returned. During the fighting, though, some Aztec warriors were infected with smallpox. The disease soon swept across Mexico, killing Montezuma and 3 million Mexican Indians, about one-third of Mexico's total population. Because most Spanish soldiers had survived smallpox in Europe, they did not become ill. A Spanish priest described the frightful event: "As the [Mexican] Indians did not know the remedy of the disease . . . they died in heaps, like bedbugs. In many places it happened that everyone in a house died and, as it was impossible to bury the great number of dead, they pulled down the houses over them so that their homes became their tombs."[13]

Meanwhile, Cortés reorganized his army and returned to Tenochtitlán in 1521. Cortés easily defeated the weakened Aztec army and paved the way for the Spanish conquest of Mexico. The mighty Aztec Empire had been vanquished by smallpox and would never rise again.

From Mexico, smallpox spread south through Central America to South America, where it reached the vast empire of the Inca. At its height, the Incan Empire extended along the west coast of South America, from modern Ecuador to central Chile. Historians estimate that between 3.5 and 16 million Indians, from various tribes, occupied this region. The Incan capital was Cuzco, located high in the Andes Mountains in what is now Peru. A smallpox epidemic struck Cuzco and the surrounding area in 1527. The Incan emperor Huayna Capac and about one hundred thousand others, including the nation's highest military and political leaders, were killed. The emperor died before he could name a successor, which resulted in a fierce rivalry for the throne between his sons, Huáscar and Atahualpa. Civil war followed, from which Atahualpa emerged as the Incan ruler in 1532.

Soon afterward, the Spanish conqueror Francisco Pizarro invaded the Incan Empire. With the advantages of guns, horses, and artillery, Pizarro conquered Atahualpa and took over the Inca and their land, which was rich in gold, silver, and other minerals. The Inca, struck by another smallpox epidemic, were unable to regroup and expel the Spaniards. A Spanish observer wrote,

> [The Inca] died by the scores and hundreds. . . . Corpses were scattered over the fields or piled up in the houses or huts. . . . The fields were uncultivated; the herds were untended; and the workshops and mines were without laborers. . . . The price of food rose to such an extent that many persons found it beyond their reach. They escaped the foul disease, only to be wasted by famine. [14]

Once again, a great empire had been felled by smallpox.

Christian missionaries, who followed European explorers to the New World, were also partially responsible for the ravages of smallpox among the Indians. In the 1500s, Jesuit missionaries began to arrive in Brazil along with Portuguese settlers. The missionaries persuaded Brazilian Indians to live in settlements, where they would be baptized and live as Christians. By the middle of the seventeenth century, more than one hundred thousand Indians were crowded around ten Jesuit missions in Brazil. A smallpox epidemic in 1660 spread through the packed colonies and killed about forty-four thousand Indians. Another outbreak in 1669 slew twenty thousand more. As their converts died, the Jesuits brought in more Indians from the interior, resulting in mass slaughter by smallpox. John Hemming, an Englishman who wrote about the conquest of the Brazilian Indians, commented, "Some of the Jesuits may have believed that it was better for Indians to be baptized but dead than heathen but alive and free." [15]

The situation was similar in late-eighteenth-century Mexico. The Spanish, who controlled Mexico, compelled many Mexican Indians to live in Catholic missions, accept Christianity, and submit to Spanish control. Mission settlements, with large populations in confined areas, were repeatedly struck by smallpox. In addition to killing vast numbers of people, the plague wreaked havoc on local Indian culture. Too few Indians were left to farm and provide food; family ties were disrupted; religious ceremonies were neglected; and friends and relatives of victims fled.

Native Americans Are Ravaged by the Scourge

Like their neighbors to the south, North American Indians were ravaged by smallpox. The scourge began in the 1600s, when colonists from Great Britain, France, and Holland arrived in North America, bringing smallpox and other diseases. The first smallpox epidemic in the region occurred in the eastern part of the continent. In 1633, an outbreak struck Algonquian Indians living near the Plymouth Colony in Massachusetts. Some colonists believed that God afflicted the Indians with smallpox. Years later, Increase Mather, one of Boston's leading Puritan clergymen from 1664 to 1723, wrote about the incident:

Increase Mather, a Puritan clergyman living in Boston, documented the first outbreak of smallpox in North America.

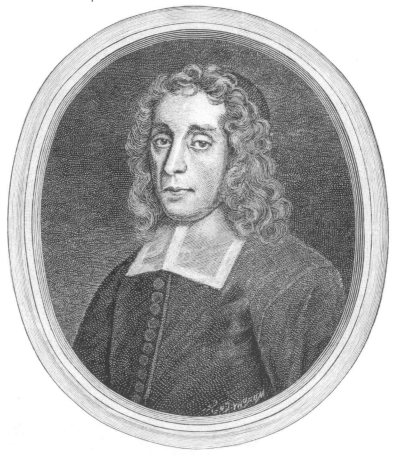

The Indians began to be quarrelsome concerning the bounds of the land they had sold to the English, but God ended the controversy by sending the smallpox amongst the Indians . . . who were before that exceeding numerous. Whole towns of them were swept away, in some of them not so much as one Soul escaping the destruction. [16]

Smallpox soon spread to other Indian tribes, with appalling consequences. The governor of Canada described a 1679 outbreak among the Iroquois of what is now upper New York State and Canada: "The small pox desolates them to such a degree, that they think no longer of meeting nor of wars, but only of bewailing the dead, of whom there is already an immense number." [17]

North American colonists, many of whom had survived smallpox in Europe, were not affected as severely as the native population. However, they suffered from smallpox, too. In Boston alone, there were six major outbreaks between 1636 and 1698, and a massive epidemic in 1721.

Trading Posts Become Smallpox Dispersal Centers

Trading posts, where Native Americans exchanged furs for manufactured goods, were unintentional dispersal stations for smallpox. By 1770, Britain's Hudson's Bay Company had seven fur-trading houses in east-central Canada, the region inhabited by the Plains Indians. Historians speculate that the smallpox virus made its way from Mexico City to New Orleans and then traveled up the Mississippi and Missouri Rivers to the Plains region. There, it caused an epidemic that raged from 1779 to 1783. Indians infected with smallpox began to appear at the Hudson House trading post, on the North Saskatchewan River, in October 1781. Mitchell Oman, an employee of Hudson House, noted the misery of the local Indians: "They were in such a state of despair and despondence, that they could hardly converse with us." [18] Native Americans traveling from one trading post to another quickly spread the disease, and by 1782, tribes throughout the region were affected. A worker at the York Factory trading post, near the Nelson and Hayes rivers, wrote, "Hundreds [of Indians] lay expiring together without assistance, or the least glimmering hopes of recovery." [19]

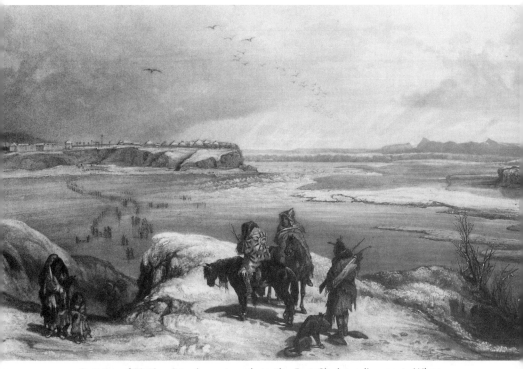

A group of Native Americans travels to the Fort Clark trading post. When Indians came to Fort Clark to obtain manufactured goods they were sometimes unintentionally infected with smallpox.

Half a century later, Native American tribes in the western territories (now the northern United States) were almost wiped out by another smallpox epidemic, which seethed from 1837 to 1840. In the 1800s, American Great Plains Indians were divided among nomadic tribes—such as the Sioux, Assiniboin, Blackfoot, and Gros Ventres—and tribes with permanent settlements—such as the Arikara, Hidatsa, and Mandan. All the tribes exchanged goods at trading posts.

Fort Clark, in what is now North Dakota, was the main trading post for the Mandan Indians. In June 1837, the American Fur Company's steamboat, the *St. Peter,* arrived at Fort Clark carrying a crew member with smallpox. The Indians came to Fort Clark to get manufactured goods and left carrying the smallpox virus. The disease quickly spread through the Mandan tribe, causing enormous misery and death. In August 1837, the post commander, F.A. Chardon, noted, "The Mandans are dying, 8–10 everyday. An old fellow lost the whole of his family to the number of 14 today." [20] The two Mandan villages, on the banks of the Missouri River, were destroyed by the disease. George Catlin, an artist who studied and painted Midwestern tribes, wrote, "There was but one continual crying and howling and praying to the Great Spirit for his protection. . . . Nobody thought of burying the dead. Whole families together were left in horrid and loathsome piles in their own wigwams, with a few buffalo robes thrown over them, there to decay, and be devoured by their own dogs." [21] Of the sixteen hundred Mandan Indians, only thirty-one survived.

Trading vessels soon carried smallpox farther north to Fort Union, where it infected the Assiniboin, and Fort McKenzie, where it struck the Blackfoot Indians. Both tribes suffered enormous losses from the disease. This pattern was repeated again and again, as smallpox infected one tribe after another.

From the region of the upper Missouri River, smallpox spread to Indians across the continent, including the Sioux, Gros Ventres, Crow, Pawnee, Osage, Kiowa, Chickasaw, Choctaw, and Comanche. Historians estimate that one hundred thousand to three hundred thousand Native Americans died during the nineteenth-century outbreak. In an unsigned letter dated June 6, 1838, an American observer wrote, "We have, from the trading posts on the . . . Missouri [River], the most frightful accounts of the ravages of the small pox among the Indians. The number of the victims within a few months is estimated at 30,000, and the pestilence is still spreading. . . . In whatever direction we go, we see nothing but melancholy wrecks of human life." [22]

Natives of the New World were struck especially hard by smallpox because they had no immunity to the disease and no way to prevent it. By the 1700s, however, a crude method of controlling smallpox, called inoculation, was spreading through the Old and New Worlds.

Chapter 3

Inoculation to Prevent Epidemics

BY THE BEGINNING of the eighteenth century, smallpox had killed countless people and was a constant threat in the world's major cities. British historian Thomas Babington Macaulay wrote in his *History of England*, "The smallpox was always present, filling the churchyard with corpses, tormenting with constant fears all whom it had not yet stricken, leaving on those whose lives it spared the hideous traces of its power, turning the babe into a changeling at which the mother shuddered, and making the eyes and cheeks of a betrothed maiden objects of horror to the lover."[23]

Communities used quarantine to control the spread of smallpox. This required isolating infected individuals to keep them from transmitting the disease. Smallpox patients were housed in secluded facilities such as "smallpox ships" moored in harbors or "pesthouses" far from population centers. Smallpox victims stayed in these grim, dirty places until they either died or recovered. Quarantine provided only temporary protection to those who were not immune to the disease, however, because people who avoided infection during one epidemic might get sick during a later outbreak. Thus, urban dwellers sought a better way to control smallpox.

Inoculation Spreads to Great Britain

In the early 1700s, reports of the ancient custom of inoculation—used in China, India, Russia, North Africa, Turkey, and the Middle East—reached England. Inoculation, also called variolation, involved purposely infecting people with a *mild* form of smallpox.

Inoculated individuals became ill but developed few pustules and little scarring. Moreover, inoculated people usually recovered, and after recovering they were immune to the disease. Though it was not understood at the time, individuals who survived smallpox developed lifelong antibodies (substances that destroy germs) against the Variola virus that causes the illness.

Methods of inoculation differed from place to place. In China, the practice involved grinding up smallpox scabs from mild cases and then blowing the powder up the noses of susceptible people. In India, small cuts were made in the skin, and scabs or pus from smallpox pustules was inserted into the slits. In Russia, people were slapped with branches that had previously been used on smallpox victims. In Turkey, susceptible people had a vein punctured or an arm scraped and then smallpox matter was introduced with a needle. No matter which procedure was used, inoculation lowered the risk of dying from smallpox. Overall, the death rate was reduced from about 30 percent for people who acquired the disease naturally to 1 or 2 percent for individuals inoculated with mild forms of smallpox.

Lady Mary Wortley Montagu, a writer and poet and the wife of the British ambassador to Turkey, had smallpox as a young woman. She survived but was left badly scarred and without eyelashes. Having suffered through the disease, Lady Montagu was interested when she observed inoculation in Constantinople, Turkey, in 1717. In a letter to an English friend, Lady Montagu wrote,

> The small-pox, so fatal, and so general amongst us, is here entirely harmless, by the invention of *ingrafting* [inoculation], which is the term they give it. There is a set of old women, who make it their business to perform the operation, every autumn in the month of September, when the great heat is abated. People send to one another to know if any of their family has a mind to have the small-pox: they make parties for this purpose, and when they are met (commonly fifteen or sixteen together), the old woman comes with a nut-shell full of the matter of the best sort of small-pox, and asks what vein you please to have opened. . . . Every year thousands undergo

this operation: and the French Ambassador says pleasantly that they take the small-pox here by way of diversion, as they take the waters in other countries. [24]

To protect her children, Lady Montagu had her physician—Dr. Charles Maitland—inoculate her five-year-old son, Edward, in Constantinople in 1718 and her four-year-old daughter, Mary, in

Lady Montagu encouraged smallpox inoculation throughout England, and even recommended the procedure to Britain's Royal Palace.

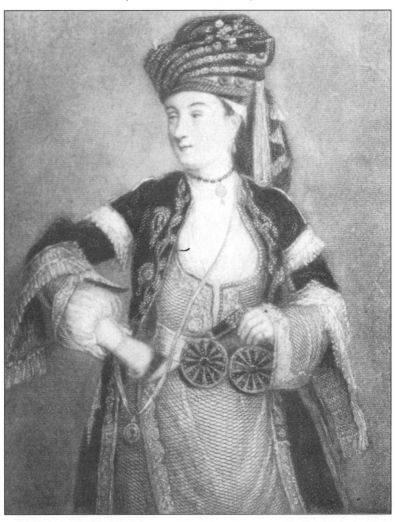

London in 1721. Mary's inoculation was written up in London newspapers and acclaimed as a complete success.

Lady Montagu encouraged inoculation in England and recommended the technique to the British royal family. This shocked some people. English physician Dr. William Wagstaffe wrote, "Posterity will scarcely be brought to believe that a method practiced only by a few ignorant women, amongst an illiterate and unthinking people, should on a sudden, and upon slender experience . . . be received into the Royal Palace."[25] To suppress dissent, Prince George and Princess Caroline (the prince and princess of Wales) decided to test the procedure. During a smallpox epidemic in 1721, they had Dr. Maitland inoculate six condemned prisoners in London's Newgate Prison. The procedure was closely observed by the king's physician, Sir Hans Sloane, and twenty-five members of the Royal Society and the College of Physicians. The inoculated convicts, promised freedom if they pulled through, all survived. The experiment was repeated on six orphan boys, who also survived. Finally, the princess of Wales had her two daughters, Amelia and Caroline, inoculated.

Once inoculation was accepted by the royal family, it quickly spread across England. Despite this, many doctors, ministers, and others furiously objected to the technique. Some feared that mildly ill patients would travel around, spreading smallpox through the community. Others thought that to protect oneself from deadly smallpox was to go against God's will. In 1772, the Reverend Edward Massey preached a sermon titled "The Dangerous and Sinful Practice of Inoculation," in which he declared "that diseases are sent by Providence for the punishment of sin; and that the proposed attempt to prevent them is a diabolical operation."[26]

Nevertheless, Lady Montagu encouraged physicians to perform inoculations and wrote letters to newspapers supporting the practice. By 1723, inoculation was fairly common in England, especially among wealthy citizens who were able to afford it. And it was not long before doctors all over Europe were learning the technique and performing inoculations.

American Colonists Are Inoculated

Cotton Mather, son of the clergyman Increase Mather (who once preached that God afflicted Indians with smallpox to help English settlers), served as pastor of North Church in Boston, Massachusetts, from 1685 to 1728. In the early 1700s, Cotton Mather heard about inoculation from his African slave, Onesimus. Onesimus described an operation that had given him "something of ye smallpox"[27] that would always protect him from the disease. Mather, interested in medicine, investigated the procedure. Then, when a smallpox epidemic struck Boston in 1721, Mather called for doctors to inoculate Boston residents.

One Boston physician, Dr. Zabdiel Boylston, responded to Mather's request. Boylston began by inoculating his six-year-old son, Thomas, and two African slaves. Many Boston residents were outraged. As in England, some objected on religious grounds. Others feared that inoculation would spread the disease. One furious person threw a homemade grenade into Mather's house. A note on the grenade read, "Cotton Mather, you dog. Damn you! I'll inoculate you with this, and a pox to you!"[28] Other angry Bostonians threatened to drag Dr. Boylston out and hang him.

In truth, there was good reason for concern. Inoculated people were expected to remain isolated for several weeks, to avoid spreading the disease. Some thoughtless individuals, however, went about their daily business—working, visiting, shopping, attending church, and so on—which dispersed

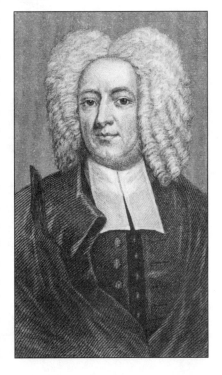

Cotton Mather supported the first smallpox inoculations in the New World.

the illness and triggered new outbreaks. Nevertheless, dread of the expanding smallpox epidemic induced many Bostonians to accept inoculation. By the end of the outbreak, in the spring of 1722, Dr. Boylston and two colleagues had inoculated 280 patients. Only six of them—about 2 percent—died from smallpox. This compared well with the 5,800 citizens who acquired smallpox naturally, of whom 844—approximately 15 percent—perished.

Inoculation was introduced to Philadelphia, New York City, and Charleston, South Carolina, in the 1730s, when epidemics struck those cities. The procedure remained very controversial, however. Thus, some colonies allowed inoculation only during epidemics and

Benjamin Franklin, pictured here working in his print shop, urged authorities to make smallpox inoculation available to the lower classes as well as the rich.

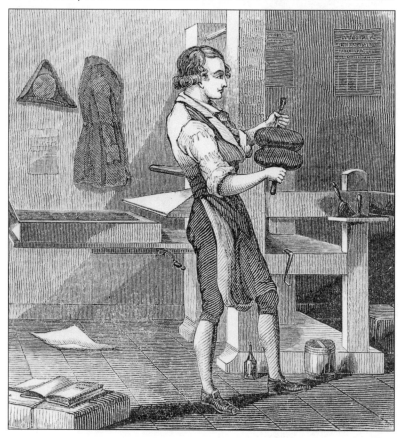

imposed strict quarantines on inoculated individuals. Nevertheless, physicians set up "inoculation hospitals" in many cities. These large, moneymaking clinics charged high fees and were usually patronized by the wealthy. As elsewhere, affluent families often made inoculation into a social event. Relatives or groups of friends got together to be inoculated and remained together for the entire isolation period. Poor working people, most of whom could not afford inoculation, became the main victims of smallpox in the American colonies.

Benjamin Franklin, then editor of the *Pennsylvania Gazette,* highlighted the plight of the lower classes. He wrote, "The expense of having the operation [inoculation] performed by a surgeon has been pretty high in some parts of America." For a tradesman with a large family, for example, "it amounts to more money than he can well spare."[29] Moreover, most laborers could not afford to miss work for three to four weeks, the length of the quarantine period. Franklin and others urged authorities to make inoculation available to the poor as well as the rich. As a result, Philadelphia founded the Society for the Inoculation of the Poor in 1774. By the end of the 1700s, the efforts of the society and similar organizations had greatly lowered the death rate of colonists in America from smallpox.

Biological Warfare Against Native Americans

Native Americans, dispersed across the North American continent, were left out of inoculation programs. In fact, British forces intentionally spread smallpox among Native Americans in the first recorded use of biological warfare.

In 1763, during the French and Indian War, a confederation of tribes led by the Ottawa chief Pontiac attempted to drive the British out of the Midwest and Great Lakes region. Sir Jeffrey Amherst, commander-in-chief of the British forces in North America, was enraged by the Indian attacks. In a letter to Colonel Henry Bouquet, the officer in charge of subduing the Pontiac rebellion, Amherst suggested, "Could it not be contrived to send the smallpox among those disaffected tribes of Indians? We must, on this occasion, use every stratagem in our power to reduce them."[30] Bouquet wrote back, asking Amherst whether he should give contaminated blankets to the Indians. Amherst consented, and Colonel Bouquet replied, "I will try to [infect] the [Indians] by means of some blankets that may fall in their hands, taking care however not to get the disease myself." [31] Amherst, who wanted to wipe out the Indians, wrote back: "You will do well to [infect] the Indians by means of blankets as well as to try every other method that can serve to extirpate [destroy] this execrable [detestable] race." [32]

Bouquet relayed this plan to Captain Simeon Ecuyer, who arranged a meeting with Native American chiefs at Fort Pitt in western Pennsylvania. William Trent, an officer who attended the meeting, wrote that the soldiers had given the Indians "two blankets and an handkerchief out of the small pox hospital," and noted, "I hope it will have the desired effect." [33] Historians do not know whether this plan succeeded, although a smallpox epidemic did break out among the nearby Ohio Indians a few months later.

Inoculation During the American Revolution

Although inoculation was spreading through American colonies, most of the American army was not inoculated. Thus, when the American Revolution began, smallpox was a much bigger problem for American-born troops than for British troops. Most British soldiers had either survived smallpox or been inoculated and thus were immune. The majority of American troops, however, were susceptible to the disease.

When General George Washington became commander-in-chief of the Continental Army in 1775, smallpox was widespread across North America. General Washington, who had survived smallpox as a young man, was concerned about his soldiers. He had good reason to worry, as smallpox was rampant in battle zones like Massachusetts and Quebec.

In June 1775, General Washington and his forces surrounded Boston, trapping British troops, as well as American patriots, in the city. Boston was in the grip of a smallpox epidemic, and hordes of people were dying. Fearing that his men would become infected, Washington kept individuals with smallpox away from the Continental Army. In a letter to Congress dated July 1775, Washington wrote, "I have been particularly attentive to the least symptom of the smallpox: and hitherto we have been so fortunate as to have

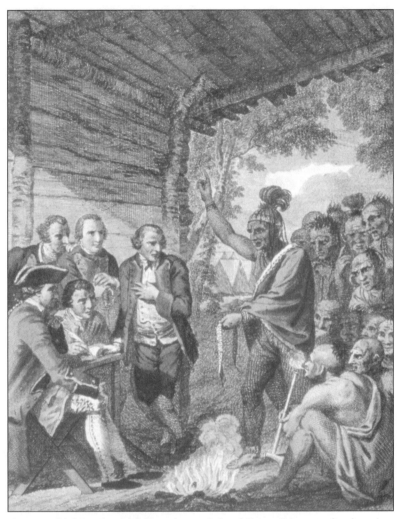

Ottawa chief Pontiac (right) confronts Colonel Henry Bouquet after learning that British forces had intentionally infected Indians with smallpox.

every person removed, so soon as noting [symptoms], to prevent any communication, but I am most apprehensive it may gain in the camps. We shall continue the utmost vigilance against this dangerous enemy."[34] Washington did not permit his troops to be inoculated. He thought inoculated soldiers might spread the disease while they were infectious, and he did not want to diminish the army's ranks by quarantining inoculated men.

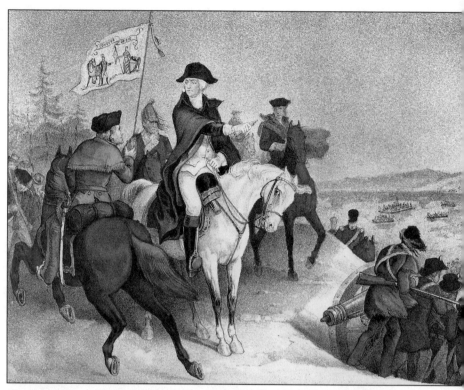

During the siege of Boston, General George Washington (on white horse) was concerned that the British would use the smallpox virus as a biological weapon.

As the siege of Boston continued, General Washington grew fearful that British officers might try to infect American troops by permitting smallpox sufferers to leave the city. In December 1775, General Washington wrote to Congress once again: "The information I received that the enemy intended spreading smallpox among us I could not suppose them capable of. I now must give some credit to it as it made its appearance on several of those [refugees] who last came out of Boston."[35] When British officers finally surrendered Boston in March 1776, Washington at first allowed only one thousand American troops who had already had smallpox to enter the city. He did not want susceptible soldiers infected by any contaminated objects the British had left behind. Still, the danger of smallpox increased as Bostonians, now free to travel, spread the disease.

Smallpox was also a factor in Revolutionary War battles around Quebec. In the fall of 1775, General Richard Montgomery and Colonel Benedict Arnold assembled more than three thousand Continental troops outside Quebec, which was then under British control. The officers hoped to free Quebec from British rule and add it to American territory. Like other parts of North America, Quebec was in the midst of a smallpox epidemic. The dreaded disease soon spread to the American troops, striking down one soldier after another.

The Continental officers led their diminished forces into Quebec on December 31, 1775. The assault failed completely. General Montgomery and about fifty soldiers were killed, Colonel Arnold was wounded, four hundred soldiers were captured, and the rest of the American troops were driven back. The remaining Continental forces resumed their blockade of Quebec, but their ranks continued to shrink from disease, desertion, and completed tours of duty.

By the beginning of May 1776, only nineteen hundred American soldiers remained, nearly half of them suffering from smallpox. Thus, when British reinforcements arrived later in the month, the Continental soldiers abandoned their positions and fled. The British found numerous sick men left behind, many unable to walk.

George Washington Has American Troops Inoculated

The dreadful incidents at Boston and Quebec—and the fear that the British would use smallpox as a weapon—convinced General George Washington to order the inoculation of Continental soldiers. In January 1777, General Washington wrote the medical director of the army: "Finding the smallpox to be spreading much, and fearing no precaution can prevent it from running through the whole of our army, I have determined that the troops shall be inoculated. . . . I would fain hope . . . that in a short space of time we shall have an army that is not subject to this the greatest of calamities that can befall it." [36] Inoculation programs were soon under way in Connecticut, Maryland, New Jersey, New York, Pennsylvania, and Virginia.

The American Revolution ended when the British surrendered at Yorktown, Virginia, in October 1781. Historian Hugh Thursfield summed up the influence of inoculation on the Revolutionary War:

> I do not, of course, ignore the many other factors which enabled the American colonists to secure their independence . . . but I think it is fair to claim that an intelligent and properly controlled application of the only method [inoculation] then known of defeating the ravages of smallpox, which in the years 1775–1776 threatened to ruin the American cause, was a factor of considerable importance in the eventual outcome of the War of Independence.[37]

British officers surrender their arms at Yorktown. Smallpox inoculation greatly contributed to the American victory in the Revolutionary War.

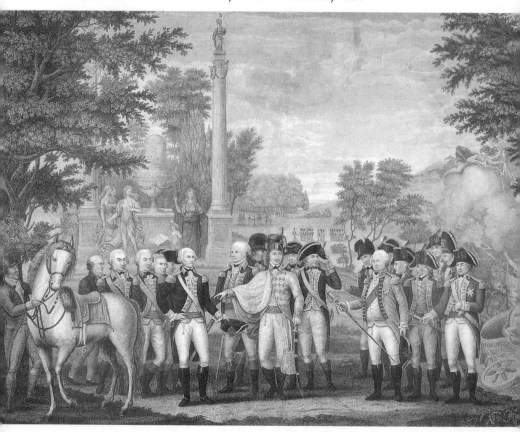

The Scourge Continues

Inoculation greatly diminished, but did not eliminate, smallpox outbreaks in America. Many southern soldiers, as well as colonists and Native Americans, remained uninoculated. This was due both to the expense of the procedure and to the fact that many people fiercely opposed inoculation. When smallpox struck Salem, North Carolina, in April 1779, a community of Moravians (evangelical Protestants) considered inoculation. Nearby settlers violently protested, however, fearing that the procedure might spread the disease. One of the Moravians angrily commented, "Our ignorant and malicious neighbors threatened to destroy the town if we inoculated, so the smallpox stayed among us until October." [38]

Over time, as inoculation became more available and increasingly accepted, fewer deaths were caused by smallpox. By the end of the 1700s, however, a better way to control the disease—vaccination—was about to sweep the world.

Chapter 4

The Smallpox Vaccine Is Developed

I N THE LATE 1700s, as inoculation became more common in Europe and America, the death rate from smallpox declined. Epidemics still broke out, though, with large cities being hit especially hard. The majority of victims were poor people, most of whom had not been inoculated. This started to change after a young country doctor named Edward Jenner developed a vaccine that would bring the scourge under control at last.

Young Edward Jenner

Edward Jenner was born in 1749 in Berkeley, a town in the English county of Gloucestershire. Jenner's parents died when he was five, and his older brother, Stephen, raised him. When a smallpox epidemic struck Gloucestershire in 1757, Jenner and several other children were inoculated by a local pharmacist. The pharmacist's technique, common at the time, was long and uncomfortable. First, he prepared the children by bleeding them many times over six weeks and giving them laxatives to empty their stomachs. The pharmacist then scratched each child's arm with a knife and fastened a dried smallpox scab over the wound. Jenner and the other children stayed with the pharmacist for several weeks, until they were no longer infectious. Once Jenner returned home, he still needed another month to fully recover from the illness, the bleedings, and the laxatives.

Even as a child, Edward Jenner was interested in nature and science. Thus, when he was thirteen, his brother apprenticed him to Dr. Daniel Ludlow, a physician. During his time with Ludlow, Jenner overheard milkmaids and farmers say that they could not get smallpox because they had already had cowpox, a mild disease that afflicts cattle. Cattle with cowpox developed pustules on their udders and teats. Farmworkers often acquired cowpox by milking infected animals. The farmers got sores ("milkers' nodules") on their hands, which quickly healed.

When Jenner was twenty-one, he became a medical student at St. George's Hospital in London, where he studied under the famous physician and scientist Dr. John Hunter. Dr. Hunter educated Jenner in anatomy, medicine, and surgical techniques. Even more important, Hunter taught Jenner the value of scientific research. "Why think," Dr. Hunter would say, "why not try the experiment?"[39] Later, Jenner used the experimental approach to prove his theories about smallpox vaccine.

Jenner finished his medical studies in 1773, opened an office in his hometown of Berkeley, and became a country doctor. When

Cowpox sores blister the hand of Sarah Nelmes, an English milkmaid. Using material from her wounds, Edward Jenner experimented with using cowpox as an immunization against smallpox.

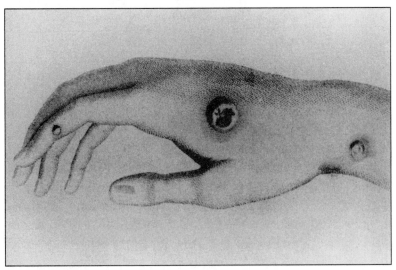

smallpox outbreaks struck Gloucestershire, Jenner traveled around the county, inoculating people. Jenner knew that inoculation was somewhat risky and that a small percentage of inoculated people died from smallpox. He also noted that some patients could not be successfully inoculated. That is, they did not develop the expected "mild smallpox," or any other illness, following inoculation. Upon investigation, Jenner learned that these individuals had previously had cowpox. Such observations, combined with farmworkers' stories about cowpox protecting them from smallpox, led Jenner to believe that deliberately inoculating people with cowpox would immunize them against smallpox. Moreover, cowpox inoculations would be safer than smallpox inoculations since cowpox is a mild, nonfatal disease.

Jenner Develops Smallpox Vaccine

Jenner wanted to test his theory. However, cowpox was a fleeting disease. It appeared only in certain parts of England and only at rare intervals. Because of this, Jenner decided to try to transfer cowpox from one human being to another.

On May 14, 1796, Jenner inoculated an eight-year-old boy, James Phipps, with cowpox material from a milkmaid, Sarah Nelmes. The boy developed cowpox and quickly recovered. Jenner, who examined Phipps every day, observed, "On the ninth day, he became a little chilly, lost his appetite, and had a headache. . . . [He] spent the night with some degree of restlessness, but on the day following he was perfectly well."[40]

On July 1, Jenner inoculated Phipps with smallpox material. As expected, the boy did not get sick. On July 19, Jenner happily wrote a friend: "But now listen to the most delightful part of my story. The boy has since been inoculated for the smallpox which as I ventured to predict produced no [ill] effects [whatsoever]. I shall now pursue my experiments with redoubled ardor."[41] Jenner repeated the experiment with several other patients—including his eleven-month-old son, Robert—with great success. Later, scientists learned that this procedure works because cowpox viruses are very closely related to smallpox viruses. Thus, people injected with cowpox produce antibodies that destroy both cowpox and smallpox viruses.

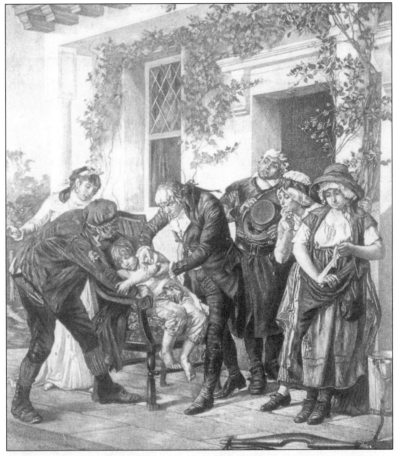

Jenner (center) inoculates young James Phipps in 1796. The experiment was a success and led to the creation of the smallpox vaccine.

With his experiment, Jenner demonstrated not only that cowpox protected people from smallpox but also that cowpox could be transferred from one individual to another. This was vital, because person-to-person transmission would be required to provide a constant supply of vaccine in the absence of naturally occurring cowpox.

Jenner Champions Vaccination

Jenner believed he had developed a safe method of preventing smallpox. He described his findings in a pamphlet titled *An Inquiry into the Causes and Effects of the Variolae Vaccinae, a Disease Discovered in Some of the Western Counties of England, Particularly Gloucestershire, and Known by the Name of Cowpox,* published in 1798. Jenner called the cowpox inoculation matter "vaccine," from *vacca,* the Latin word for "cow." He named the inoculation procedure "vaccination." Today, the words *vaccine* and *vaccination* are used for all substances and procedures that confer immunity to all kinds of diseases.

Jenner continued to refine his procedure, stating, "I shall myself continue to prosecute this inquiry, encouraged by the pleasing hope of its becoming essentially beneficial to mankind." [42] Jenner wanted the poor, as well as the rich, to have access to vaccination.

Edward Jenner poses for a nineteenth-century portrait. Jenner championed smallpox vaccination, which he often provided free of charge to the poor.

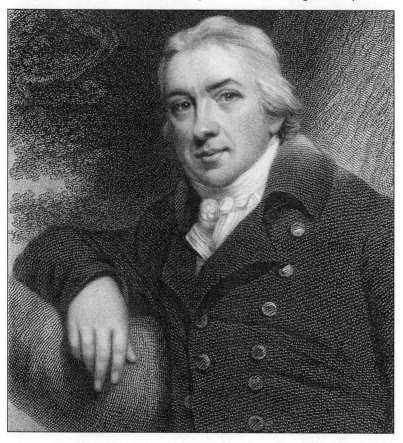

So he periodically provided free vaccination to people in Gloucestershire. Jenner's friend John Baron noted, "[Jenner] offered gratuitous [vaccination] to all the poor who thought fit to apply at stated periods. . . . These benevolent invitations were, in the main very generally accepted, parents bringing their children in great numbers both from the town and adjoining parishes."[43]

Jenner devised a way to preserve dried cowpox matter on quills, thread, slivers of ivory, and in glass tubes so that he could supply his vaccine to other doctors. He did this both to encourage vaccination and to guarantee the use of carefully chosen vaccine. Jenner knew that pustules on the udders of infected cows differed. Although all were called "cowpox" and all could infect humans, only one kind provided protection against smallpox. Jenner called this type "true cowpox." Even true cowpox, however, conferred immunity to smallpox only when matter was taken from fresh pustules.

Although many physicians were perform' g inoculations, not everyone in England had the opportunity t be vaccinated by a doctor. Therefore, some people obtained cow ox material and performed vaccinations themselves. Powell Snell, a friend of Jenner's, observed, "The housewife scratched with her needle, the cobbler with his awl, and even shepherd boys inoculate[d] each other with their pocket knives."[44] This practice, which sometimes led to infection, endangered people's lives, and—when performed with spurious vaccine—provided no protection from smallpox.

Even vaccinations done by doctors had tragic consequences when ineffective or contaminated vaccine was used. In 1799, for example, a smallpox outbreak in England was traced to two London physicians, Dr. William Woodville at St. Pancras Smallpox Hospital and Dr. George Pearson, director of an independent vaccination program. Unwilling to wait for Jenner's carefully selected vaccine, the doctors obtained their own cowpox matter from infected animals at London dairies. The physicians used the vaccine, followed by the person-to-person technique, to vaccinate several hundred people. Unfortunately, at some point the cowpox matter became contaminated with virulent smallpox matter, causing many illnesses and at least one death.

Vaccinations continued, however, and by 1801 more than one hundred thousand people in England had been successfully vaccinated against smallpox.

Vaccination Spreads to the United States

Soon after Jenner's *Variolae Vaccinae* pamphlet was published, it was translated into Dutch, French, German, Latin, and Spanish, and his technique spread to Europe, North America, South America, and Asia. Dr. Louis Sacco, who performed vaccinations in Italy, wrote Jenner in 1800: "It is to the Genius of Medicine, and the favorite child of nature that I have the honor to write. The name of Jenner will always be beloved by all posterity. . . . May you live, my dear sir, a long while for the good of humanity." [45]

The first vaccinations in the United States were performed by Dr. Benjamin Waterhouse, a professor at Harvard Medical School in Cambridge, Massachusetts. After studying Jenner's publications, Waterhouse was excited by the Englishman's discovery. In 1800, Waterhouse wrote, "On perusing this work, I was struck with the unspeakable advantages that might accrue to this country, and indeed to the human race at large, from the discovery of a mild distemper [disease] that would ever after secure the constitution from that terrible scourge, the small pox." [46] Waterhouse resolved to test the technique himself. In the summer of 1800, he vaccinated his four children, Daniel, Benjamin, Mary, and Elizabeth, and two servants, Samuel Carter and Kesiah Flag. When the children and servants were subsequently inoculated with smallpox, they did not become ill. Encouraged by these results, and wishing "to convince the faithless, and silence the mischievous," [47] Waterhouse vaccinated additional New England residents. He published his findings in newspaper articles and in a pamphlet titled *A Prospect of Exterminating the Small Pox.*

Attempts to Control the Devouring Monster

Once Waterhouse was convinced that vaccination prevented smallpox, a disease he called the "devouring monster," [48] he began a campaign to promote the procedure in America. At first, Waterhouse tried to control the distribution of the vaccine himself, supplying doctors with cowpox matter in exchange for 25 percent of their profits or a flat fee of $150. In addition to benefiting financially, Waterhouse wanted to ensure the use of "genuine" vaccine to avoid mistakes like those that had occurred in England. Waterhouse published many pamphlets and newspaper articles warning people of the dangers of unregulated vaccination. Despite his efforts, though, a tragic event occurred in Marblehead, Massachusetts, in 1800. After accidentally injecting his daughter with "vaccine" that turned out to be deadly smallpox, a doctor vaccinated other people with matter from her arm. Sixty-eight people perished in the epidemic that resulted from this incident. The calamity may have occurred because, at the time, some physicians performed both inoculations and vaccinations, using the same instruments for both procedures.

Waterhouse lost exclusive control of vaccine distribution in the fall of 1800, when other physicians received vaccine supplies from Europe. So, after getting a fresh shipment of vaccine from England in 1801, Waterhouse began giving it away to local doctors. He also suggested that the Boston Board of Health establish a vaccine institution and vaccinate the poor for free.

Thomas Jefferson Helps Out

In the early 1800s, doctors across the country began to ask Waterhouse for assistance and vaccination supplies. Hence, in 1801, Waterhouse wrote to President Thomas Jefferson to ask for his help in fostering vaccination programs. Jefferson readily agreed, writing,

> Sir. I received last night, and have read with great satisfaction, your pamphlet on the subject of the kine-pock [cowpox], and pray you to accept my thanks for the communication of it. I had before attended to your publications on the subject in the newspapers, and took much interest in the result of the experiments you were making. Every friend of humanity must look with pleasure on this discovery, by which one more evil is withdrawn from the condition of man.[49]

Jefferson had eighteen members of his family and some of his neighbors vaccinated. He also helped introduce vaccination to major

American cities, including Washington, Baltimore, Philadelphia, and New York.

Jefferson tried to promote vaccination among Native Americans as well. When Chief Little Turtle led a delegation of Indians to Washington in 1801, Jefferson told them that "the Great Spirit had made a gift to the white men in showing them how to preserve themselves from the smallpox." [50] Jefferson had the Indians vaccinated by Dr. Edward Gantt and gave them vaccine to take home. Although some Indian tribes accepted vaccination, most did not. The majority of Native Americans suspected that whites wanted to harm them and take their land. Indian expert George Catlin observed, "They [Indians] see the white men urging the operation [vaccination] so earnestly they decide it must be some new . . . trick of the pale face by which they hope to gain some new advantage over them." [51]

Thomas Jefferson helped introduce smallpox vaccination to American cities as well as to some Indian tribes.

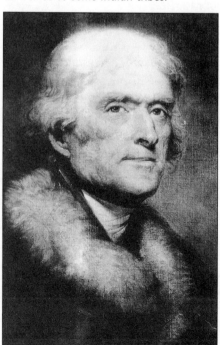

In 1832, Congress allocated money for an Indian vaccination program, but it did not succeed because the Indians did not trust the government's intentions. The situation improved with the creation of the Oregon Trail in the 1840s. White settlers, traveling along this two-thousand-mile-long overland route from Missouri to Oregon, began to flood across the country. Forts were built to protect them, and government officials—known as Indian agents—helped promote vaccination programs among Native Americans to help control smallpox in the American West.

The Royal Smallpox Expedition

Vaccination quickly spread to many countries. In the early 1800s, vaccination programs were begun in Austria, Denmark, Italy, Poland, Prussia (now part of Germany), Spain, Turkey, Russia, India, and the Middle East. Napoleon ordered the vaccination of French civilians in 1804 and French soldiers in 1805. King Charles IV of Spain launched the most ambitious vaccination program of all. In 1803, he ordered his personal physician—Dr. Francis Xavier de Balmis—to organize a royal smallpox expedition to vaccinate Spanish subjects in North America, South America, and Asia. Balmis put together a vaccination team, including himself, an assistant director named Jóse Salvany Lleopart, several medical aides, and other assistants.

The Spanish mission was an enormously difficult undertaking. Simply transporting the vaccine to people around the world was a tremendous challenge. Cowpox matter could be dried and preserved for several months, but it quickly broke down when exposed to sunlight and high temperatures. Thus, vaccine shipped across long distances often lost its potency before arrival. To overcome this obstacle, vaccine was kept "active" by transferring it from one person to another, a custom known as the arm-to-arm method.

To maintain the vaccine's effectiveness during the long sea voyage, Balmis selected twenty-two orphan boys, ages three to nine, who had never had cowpox or smallpox. During the journey to America, Balmis vaccinated the children, one after another, in a chain. Two children were vaccinated before leaving Spain, and when cowpox blisters erupted on their arms, matter from these pustules was used to vaccinate two more children. This continued until the ship arrived in Puerto Rico. To compensate the children for their services, Spanish authorities arranged for them to have foster families and schooling in the New World.

In Puerto Rico, Balmis helped establish a local "vaccination board" to monitor vaccinations. A similar board was established in each Spanish colony visited by the royal smallpox expedition. From Puerto Rico, the expedition traveled to Venezuela. There, it divided into two groups. Balmis went on to Mexico, Central America, the

Spanish Philippines, Macao, and Canton, and Salvany Lleopart remained in South America, visiting Colombia, Ecuador, Peru, Chile, and Bolivia. Each group carried cowpox matter between sealed glass plates and recruited orphan children along the way to serve as human carriers of the vaccine. Both expeditions—requiring travel by ship, horseback, boat, and mules across vast, harsh territories—were long and arduous. They were also enormously successful. In three years, the Spanish expeditions arranged for hundreds of thousands of people to be vaccinated, without charge, in villages, cities, and rural areas.

In 1806, Jenner was thrilled to receive the news about a Spanish vaccination expedition that had traveled around the world. He noted, "What a delightful narrative is here! Little did I think . . . that heaven had in store for me such abundant happiness. May I be grateful."[52]

Vaccination Replaces Inoculation

In time, vaccination replaced inoculation as the preferred method of controlling smallpox. Vaccination was easier and cheaper, since patients did not have to be quarantined for weeks at a time. Vaccination was also safer, because cowpox is not a deadly disease. These differences were noted by Henry Cline, who performed the first vaccination in London. In a 1798 letter to Jenner, Cline wrote,

> I think the substituting of cow-pox for the smallpox promises to be one of the greatest improvements that has ever been made in medicine: for it is not only so safe in itself, but also does not endanger others by contagion, in which way the small-pox has done infinite mischief. The more I think on the subject the more I am impressed with its importance.[53]

Nevertheless, there were people who vehemently disapproved of vaccination. Some opponents of vaccination felt that injecting people with "disease material" from cows was unnatural and disgusting. A critic in London wrote, "A mighty and horrible monster [named vaccination], with the horns of a bull, the hind of a horse, the jaws of a kraken [sea monster], the teeth and claws of a tiger, the tail of a cow, all the evils of Pandora's box in his belly . . . has made his appearance in the world, and devours mankind." [54] Some opponents expressed the belief that cowpox vaccinations would make people grow horns, and one woman complained that, after her daughter was vaccinated, she "coughed like a cow, and had grown hairy over her body." [55]

Others did not believe that vaccination prevented illness. One skeptic wrote, "A loathsome virus derived from the blood of a diseased brute" [56] could not prevent smallpox. Still others objected on religious grounds. In 1798, the Anti-Vaccination Society was formed by physicians and clergymen in Boston, who said that vaccination was "bidding defiance to Heaven itself, even to the will of God," and claimed that "the law of God prohibits the practice." [57]

A few people had more personal reasons for opposing vaccination. Physicians who ran inoculation clinics, for example, charged high fees and did not want to lose this lucrative source of income. Other people agreed with the economist Thomas Robert Malthus, who asserted that the human population was increasing faster than the supply of goods (food, fuel, and so on) needed to sustain it. These people argued that epidemic diseases like smallpox helped control human population growth. British surgeon John Birch, for

A satiric cartoon shows Jenner vaccinating a woman with cowpox as those already vaccinated sprout horns, hair, and even whole cows from their bodies.

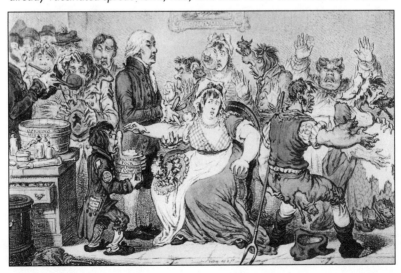

example, noted that vaccination would eliminate "a merciful means of reducing the country's poor population."[58]

Most communities, however, including a large number of religious leaders, approved of vaccination. In 1808, England established a national vaccination program, and in 1840, vaccination was ruled the only legal method of controlling smallpox in Britain. By 1821, vaccination of babies was required in Bavaria (now part of Germany), Bohemia (now part of the Czech Republic), Denmark, Norway, Russia, and Sweden. In the United States, President James Madison, in office from 1809 to 1817, signed legislation to foster vaccination. However, political differences and opposition by some doctors resulted in the repeal of the American vaccination law in 1822. Consequently, smallpox outbreaks in the United States increased once again in the mid-1800s. All in all, however, vaccination was common in many parts of the world by the middle of the 1800s.

Appreciation for Jenner

Edward Jenner received many awards for his work. He was granted honors from Harvard, Oxford, and Cambridge universities, and was made an honorary member of numerous scientific societies. He was also given financial rewards. Matthew Baillie, who entreated the British House of Commons to provide funds for Jenner, said, "In my opinion, it [vaccination] is the most important discovery ever made in medicine."[59]

Jenner also received many letters of appreciation. In 1806, President Thomas Jefferson wrote to say, "Yours is the comfortable reflection that mankind can never forget that you have lived. Future nations will know by history only that the loathsome smallpox had existed and by you has been extirpated [destroyed]."[60] The Chiefs of Five Nations in Canada, who—unlike many Indians—quickly accepted vaccination, wrote Jenner in 1807:

> Brother: Our Father [Colonel Francis Gore, lieutenant governor of upper Canada] has delivered to us the book you sent to instruct us how to use the discovery which the Great Spirit made to you whereby the smallpox, that fatal enemy of our tribe, may be driven from the earth. . . . We send with this a belt and a string of wampum in token of our appreciation of your precious gift.[61]

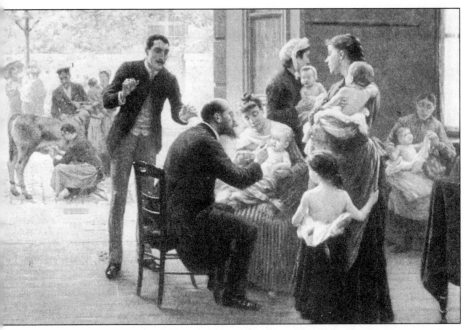

Mothers bring their babies to a doctor to receive a cowpox vaccination. In the background, an assistant extracts the cowpox virus from a cow.

Other heads of state were also grateful to Jenner. When Jenner asked the emperor Napoleon of France to release several Englishmen captured in the Napoleonic Wars, Napoleon complied, saying, "Ah, Jenner, I cannot refuse Jenner anything." [62] The king of Spain and the emperor of Austria also released English prisoners after requests by Jenner.

Vaccination Troubles

Even though Jenner's vaccination technique greatly reduced the number of deaths from smallpox in the 1800s, vaccination problems remained. This was largely because people did not yet understand how vaccine worked. Some difficulties arose from the use of ineffective "vaccines" that were not obtained from true cowpox pustules. This problem was alleviated when scientists discovered how to generate cowpox vaccine by scratching the sides of calves, inserting suitable cowpox material, and waiting for pustules to erupt. This technique provided cowpox matter that could be harvested and stored or used directly. In Italy, for example, inoculated animals were led from house to house, and children were vaccinated with matter straight from the cow. This approach spawned new difficulties, however, because animal hair and germs became mixed with the vaccine.

Contamination issues also arose with the person-to-person vaccination technique. If the vaccine passed through a person suffering from syphilis, tuberculosis, or hepatitis, for example, the germs from these diseases could be transferred along with the vaccine. This occurred in Italy in 1861, when arm-to-arm vaccination passed syphilis bacteria from a sick individual to forty-one Italian children. Englishman William Tebb, who belonged to the Anti-Vaccination League, observed, "It is not now denied by the medical profession that vaccination is [a] . . . cause of infantile [childhood] syphilis, and . . . the increase in infantile syphilis, since vaccination has been compulsory, is fourfold." [63] A similar difficulty stemmed from the use of soiled instruments. Describing vaccination aboard an English ship, Tebb said,

> The lymph [vaccine] used was of unknown origin, kept in capillary glass tubes, from whence it was blown into a cup into which the lancet [pointed instrument] was dipped. No pretense of cleaning the lancet was made; it drew blood in very many instances, and it was used upon as many as 276 during the first day. . . . No one can estimate the number of healthy, innocent children, as well as adults, who are inoculated with syphilis or other foul disease. [64]

Yet another vaccination problem arose from the fact that cowpox vaccine did not confer lifelong immunity. Since immunity waned over time, individuals sometimes contracted smallpox years after they were vaccinated. To overcome this difficulty, revaccinations, or "booster shots," were required every five to ten years. The risk that vaccination or revaccination could transfer syphilis or other illnesses, as well as the possible complications of vaccination, generated dread in some people.

Occasionally, severe—and sometimes deadly—complications were experienced by some vaccinated individuals. These side effects, caused by the live viruses in smallpox vaccine, included post-vaccinal encephalitis (virus-induced brain inflammation); progressive vaccinia (severe tissue destruction spreading from the vaccination site); eczema vaccinatum (a life-threatening skin rash); generalized vaccinia (vesicles all over the body); and accidental transfer of vaccinia viruses from the vaccination site to other parts of the body. Inadvertent infection of the eyes, for example, could result in blindness.

Smallpox Epidemics Persist

Some people refused to participate in vaccination programs, either because they feared vaccination or because they had religious objections. This, among other things, resulted in persistent smallpox epidemics in many countries. In Russia, about one hundred thousand people died from smallpox in 1856. Berlin suffered a serious epidemic in 1858, and Switzerland had three smallpox outbreaks between 1849 and 1868. Europe's worst epidemic of the nineteenth century, resulting from the Franco-Prussian War, lasted from 1870 to 1875. Historians estimate that over half a million people died from smallpox during this outbreak.

Thus, even though an effective vaccine was available, smallpox continued to plague some parts of the world until the last half of the twentieth century, when the disease was finally eradicated from the earth.

Chapter 5

Smallpox Is Eradicated

SMALLPOX CONTINUED TO plague human populations long after Edward Jenner developed the smallpox vaccine in 1796. This was due to both the reluctance of some people to be vaccinated and the difficulty of vaccinating large populations and individuals in remote regions. By the end of the nineteenth century, however, persistent vaccination programs began to eliminate smallpox from some countries. Sweden eradicated smallpox in 1895; Puerto Rico in 1899; Austria and Cuba in the 1920s; Great Britain, the Philippines, and the Soviet Union in the 1930s; and Central America, the Caribbean Islands, and the United States in the 1940s. Finally, in 1967—171 years after Jenner's great discovery—the first serious attempt to eradicate smallpox from the world began.

The Worldwide Eradication Campaign Is Launched

Smallpox had been exterminated from the United States by 1947 when a terrifying event occurred. In March of that year, an American businessman took a bus from Mexico to New York City. Upon arrival, the man felt ill and was taken to a hospital. There, he was diagnosed with severe bronchitis. The man died five days later, and doctors realized he had been suffering from smallpox. By then, the disease had spread to eleven other people, one of whom also died. The outbreak caused a near panic in New York City. In response, health authorities ordered the vaccination or revaccination of more than 6 million people, quickly stopping the spread of the disease.

Soon afterward, in 1948, the World Health Organization (WHO) was formed to improve the well-being of the earth's population.

At that time, smallpox still plagued many developing regions, especially Africa, Brazil, India, Indonesia, and Southwest Asia. In 1953, Dr. Brock Chisolm, the WHO's first director, proposed that nations undertake a global crusade to eradicate the disease. The task seemed too difficult, and the proposal was voted down.

Meanwhile, many countries continued to suffer from smallpox. In 1958, Albert Herrlich, head of the poxvirus laboratory at the University of Munich, reported a dreadful outbreak in Bombay, India. Describing the victims, he wrote,

> The head was usually covered by what appeared to be a single pustule; the nose and lips were glued together. When the tightly filled vesicles burst, the pus soaked through the bedsheet, became smeared on the blanket, and formed thick, yellowish scabs and crusts on the skin. . . . Swallowing was so painful that the patients refused all nourishment and, in spite of agonizing thirst, often also refused all fluids. . . . Wails and groans filled the rooms. . . . The patients were conscious to their last breath. Some just lay there, dull and unresponsive. They no longer shook off the flies that sat on purulent [pus-filled] eyelids, on the openings of mouth and nose, and in swarms on the inflamed areas of skin.[65]

At the 1958 World Health Assembly, Dr. Viktor M. Zhadnov, deputy minister of health of the Soviet Union, revived the proposal that the WHO attempt to eradicate smallpox. He noted that smallpox was costly to *all* nations, since even those free of the disease had to vaccinate their citizens to protect them from migrating smallpox victims. The WHO accepted the proposal in 1959, but it was not until 1966 that sufficient funds of $2.4 million for smallpox eradication were allocated. The year 1977 was set as the deadline for this goal to be achieved. Dr. Donald Ainslie Henderson, assistant chief of epidemiology at the Centers for Disease Control (CDC) in Atlanta, was chosen to lead the campaign.

In 1967, when the global eradication program began, smallpox was still common in thirty-five countries, and another forty-four countries reported smallpox victims crossing their borders. During that year, 10 to 15 million people contracted smallpox worldwide, and about 2 million died.

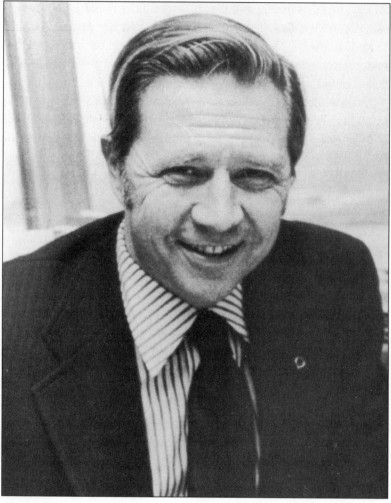

Dr. Donald Henderson led the WHO's global campaign to eradicate smallpox in 1967. That year, nearly 15 million people contracted the disease worldwide.

New Vaccines and Better Vaccination Methods Are Developed

The CDC's effort to exterminate smallpox was long and arduous, and many problems had to be overcome. One difficulty was obtaining suitable vaccines. Most smallpox vaccines being used at the time were liquids and had to be kept refrigerated. This was not possible in developing countries that had insufficient refrigeration facilities. To overcome this obstacle, the CDC started to use freeze-dried vaccines, developed by Leslie Collier in the 1950s. Freeze-dried vaccines retained their potency without refrigeration. Water was simply added to reconstitute them (restore them to usable form). However, freeze-dried vaccines from different manufacturers varied in quality and strength. Therefore, Henderson commissioned international testing centers to ensure that all vaccines met standards of safety and performance.

Soon after the smallpox vaccine was discovered, scientists and doctors began to research ways to make it more effective and less dangerous. In the 1870s, after the vaccine had been used for many years, an unusual discovery was made. The vaccine was no longer the "cowpox virus" used by Jenner but a new virus named "vaccinia." Many scientists think that, over the years, the cowpox virus mutated

Vaccinia virus particles are seen through an electron microscope. Many scientists believe that Jenner's cowpox vaccine mutated into vaccinia as it was transferred from person to person.

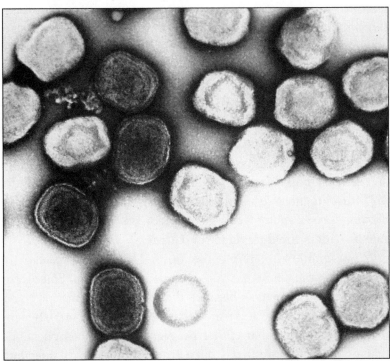

as it was transferred from person to person. Other scientists think the cowpox virus mutated in animals. However it arose, vaccinia—which is now grown in laboratories—proved to be an effective vaccine against smallpox.

Along with better vaccines, the CDC needed new methods of vaccination. The customary vaccination procedure involved placing a drop of vaccine on the recipient's arm and scratching it into the skin with a needle. This was time-consuming and did not always provide good immunity. So, the CDC experimented with "ped-o-jets," injector guns worked by foot pedals, for mass vaccinations. These worked well but were costly and required frequent maintenance. The CDC eventually turned to bifurcated needles (two-pronged needles), which were cheap and easy to use. First, the needle was dipped into a tube of vaccine to trap a drop of vaccine between the prongs. The needle was then jabbed into the recipient's arm fifteen to twenty times over a small area. The vaccination site was then covered with a loose bandage to deter the recipient from touching the area and transferring viruses to other parts of the body. Successful vaccination was demonstrated by the development of a pustule in about a week.

Locating Smallpox Outbreaks

A major hurdle to smallpox eradication was the difficulty of reaching people in remote regions. To accomplish this, Henderson recruited dedicated young workers—dubbed "virus hunters"—and sent them to countries where smallpox was rampant. There, the virus hunters assisted local health care workers. The CDC also provided jeeps, motorcycles, helicopters, and fuel so that health care providers could travel to rural areas.

However, the virus hunters found that when they reached an area, many indigenous peoples shunned vaccination. Some people avoided vaccination because they thought a smallpox god controlled the disease and feared that the god would punish them if they were vaccinated. Other people feared the complications that occasionally resulted from vaccination, such as infection,

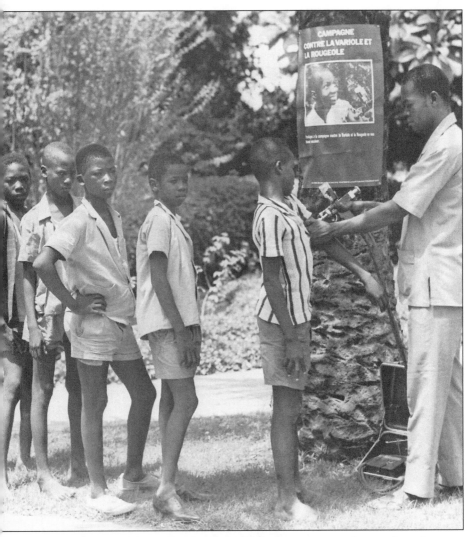

A CDC worker uses a "ped-o-jet" injector gun to vaccinate a line of young boys in a remote West African village.

blindness, or—in rare cases—death (from illnesses caused by the vaccinia virus). Thus, CDC vaccination teams were sometimes threatened with weapons or deceived. Credo Mutwa, a Zulu shaman (spiritual healer) in South Africa, remembered, "Inspectors used to come and check each child for signs of vaccination. Grains of maize would be heated up [by grandparents] and pushed against the skin of the child, and so when the school's inspectors came he saw the blisters and assumed the child had been vaccinated."[66] Some families tried to lock themselves in their houses. John Wickett, a virus hunter in India and Bangladesh, recalled, "People would lock their doors sometimes when we came by. . . . We hired these little kids to go over the walls of the homes and open the door for us from the inside. One would get in trouble for that these days but it worked, and in the end it's better to be vaccinated than to get smallpox."[67] In some towns, almost everyone hid from vaccination teams. A virus hunter who worked in southern Asia recounted, "Teams on motorcycles and Land Rovers would launch military-style raids on infected villages in Bangladesh in the middle of the night, pulling terrified men and women out from hiding places under beds, behind doors and even latrines."[68]

To locate outbreaks, CDC workers offered people rewards for reporting smallpox cases. To help villagers identify the disease, virus hunters displayed photographs of victims covered with pustules. Zafar Husain, a CDC worker in India, recalled, "In January of 1974 it was decided to try to find the whereabouts of smallpox cases during [a local fair]. . . . There was a gathering of between 10,000 to 15,000 people. . . . It was decided to fix a reward of ten rupees to anyone who would tell us about a smallpox affected village. Because of this reward system, many [affected] villages were detected."[69]

The dedication of the international virus hunters was remarkable. John Scott Porterfield, a CDC worker in Ethiopia, noted, "They never shirked their responsibilities and were fearless in carrying out their mission."[70] Many virus hunters lived in small rural towns without electricity and worked eighteen-hour days, seven days a week.

Surveillance and Containment

Until the 1960s, smallpox prevention involved mass vaccinations. Medical authorities believed that if *most* of a population was immune to smallpox, the disease would be unable to spread and would die out. This did not work in some countries, however. In India, for example, cities were so densely populated that even an 80 percent vaccination rate left many thousands of susceptible hosts. Mass vaccination also required large quantities of vaccine, which were not always available.

To overcome these problems, Dr. William Foege, working in Nigeria, developed the "surveillance and containment" strategy in 1967. Instead of mass vaccinations, the new plan called for quickly finding smallpox victims and vaccinating everyone who might come in contact with them. This created a ring of immunized people around each outbreak, which prevented the virus from spreading. Porterfield thought of these tactics as "search-and-destroy missions":

> The mind set from the epidemiologists was very clear. Find the disease, contain it, destroy it. Without question, to a person, we went, day or night, to find and fight outbreaks. . . . We vaccinated day-old babies as per order from WHO. . . . We could and did vaccinate everyone who had a left arm.[71]

By early 1972, the surveillance and containment approach had successfully eliminated smallpox from twenty African countries, as well as Brazil and Indonesia.

The End of Smallpox

The CDC continued to use the surveillance and containment strategy until smallpox was completely wiped out. The last victim of naturally occurring smallpox was twenty-three-year-old Ali Maow Maalin, a hospital cook in Merca, Somalia.

When Maalin was stricken with smallpox in October 1977, CDC workers raced to Merca. A Canadian filmmaker, Italo Costa, filmed the event, and Tod Mohamed, a health journalist, described it:

> Men, women and children were woken and coaxed or dragged outside where their faces and torsos were quickly examined— their clothing pulled away to expose the upper arm. If a shoulder lacked a circular scar, one of the strangers [virus hunters]

produced his "pitchfork"—a two-pronged needle about the length of an adult's pinkie—and dabbed it in a vial of brown liquid. Holding his captive's arm firmly, the stranger pierced the skin . . . pricking the same spot quickly about 15 or 20 times. Babies cried, old men struggled, some tried to run away. Within moments it was over and the strangers departed, continuing through Merca's darkened streets. [72]

Over the next two weeks, nearly fifty-five thousand people were vaccinated. When Maalin recovered, naturally occurring smallpox was gone from the planet.

On December 9, 1979, members of the Global Commission for the Certification of Smallpox Eradication signed a document certifying that smallpox had been eradicated from the world. When Dr. Frank Fenner, chairman of the commission, was later asked to describe the proudest moment of his life, he stated, "I suppose the single one that stands out was the day I . . . gave the short address declaring that smallpox had been eradicated globally; meaning that transmission from human to human had been stopped." [73]

Smallpox Research Continues

Although global eradication of smallpox had been accomplished, scientists and health workers became concerned about stockpiles of smallpox viruses in laboratories around the world. They feared that Variola might "escape" from a lab and cause an outbreak. Thus, in 1984, the WHO authorized only two labs to keep samples of the Variola virus: the CDC in the United States and the Institute of Virus Preparations in the former Soviet Union. The WHO ordered all other nations either to destroy their smallpox stocks or send them to the approved labs. Every country with smallpox samples agreed to comply.

In 1990, concerned that Variola might be used for biological warfare or bioterrorism, the WHO pressured the CDC and the Russian lab to destroy all smallpox stocks. The first date set for destruction was December 31, 1993. Scientists objected, however, saying they needed more time to study the virus. Researchers argued that a better understanding of Variola could help control other diseases.

They also noted that, in the event of a terrorist attack with smallpox, new antiviral drugs and new vaccines—with less dangerous side effects—would be required. To give researchers time to develop appropriate medicines and vaccines, the WHO postponed the deadline for destruction of Variola to 1995, then to 1999, then to 2002, and then indefinitely.

In 1977, CDC virus hunters raced to Somalia to examine smallpox victim Ali Maow Maalin. After Maalin was treated and fifty-five thousand additional people were vaccinated, endemic smallpox was considered extinct.

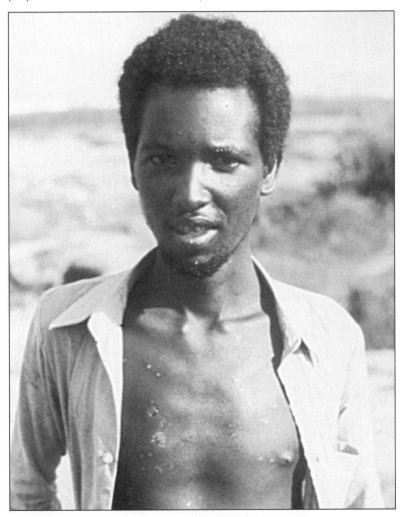

Anthrax attacks in the United States in the fall of 2001 increased fear that enemy nations or terrorist groups might use biological weapons. According to the CDC, smallpox is one of the biological agents of highest concern because it spreads easily, has a high death rate, and—in the event of an outbreak—would cause mass panic and social disruption. Thus, U.S. officials felt it was necessary to form a plan to deal with a potential smallpox attack.

Chapter 6

Smallpox as a Biological Weapon

T HE ERADICATION OF smallpox, announced in 1980, was hailed as one of humankind's greatest accomplishments. Because smallpox was no longer a threat, the World Health Organization asked all nations to stop vaccinating civilians. The United States had stopped in 1972, and all other countries ceased by 1984. However, the fear that Variola might be used as a biological weapon led a number of nations, including Australia, Canada, Israel, the Soviet Union, and the United States, to continue vaccinating their military personnel. By 1990, though, most countries had even stopped vaccinating soldiers.

The long-range consequence of these events is that *most* of the world's population is now susceptible to smallpox. Even previously vaccinated individuals may not be protected since vaccine-induced immunity declines over time. Today, there are mounting concerns in many nations that bioterrorists or outlaw countries may obtain smallpox viruses and unleash this dreadful disease. In 2001, Michael Osterholm, director of the Center for Infectious Disease Research and Policy at the University of Minnesota, wrote, "Approximately 500 million people died of smallpox in the century that just ended. . . . These staggering numbers make painfully clear how grave a global crisis any return of smallpox would represent; the use of it as a weapon would constitute the ultimate crime against humanity."[74]

A Possible Smallpox Weapon

Variola is officially confined to two laboratories, one in the United States and one in Russia, to be used for research purposes *only*.

However, in 1992, Ken Alibek, a onetime deputy director of the former Soviet Union's bioweapons program, defected to the United States. Alibek reported that beginning in 1980, his country had a secret scheme to convert Variola into a biological weapon, in violation of international law. Alibek disclosed that twenty tons of liquid smallpox had been stored at Soviet military bases, ready to be loaded into bombs or placed in warheads on intercontinental ballistic missiles.

Alibek was one of thousands of people who lost their jobs in 1992 after the breakup of the Soviet Union. At that time, Russia closed its biowarfare labs and destroyed its huge stores of liquid smallpox. Many of the displaced employees, however, were scientists and skilled laboratory technicians with access to long-lasting, freeze-dried Variola. Some of the workers may have sold their services, as well as Variola, to other countries or terrorist organizations. According to Alibek, "No one knows where they are. One can guess that they've ended up in Iraq, Syria, Libya, China, Iran, perhaps Israel, perhaps India—but no one really knows, probably not even the Russian government."[75] Some American leaders think Cuba, North Korea, Pakistan, and Serbia as well as terrorist groups like al-Qaeda and the Japanese Aum Shinrikyo cult, which released nerve gas in a Tokyo subway in 1995, may also have secret Variola stocks.

Subway passengers are raced into a hospital after a 1995 bioterrorism attack in Tokyo. American leaders believe that several countries, terrorist cells, and cults have access to smallpox stocks.

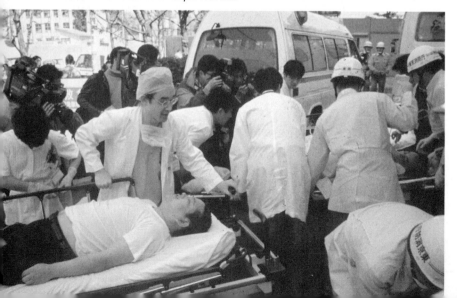

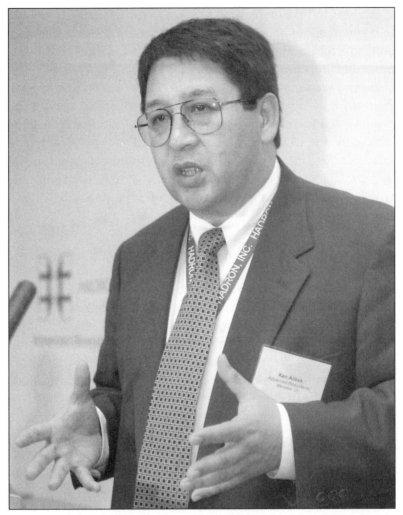

Dr. Kenneth Alibek discusses the threat of bioterrorism during a speech at George Mason University in 2001.

American officials fear that bioterrorists might release smallpox even though it would kill their own people as well as citizens of other countries. Dr. Tara O'Toole, U.S. director of the Center for Civilian Biodefense, commented, "Who knows what a terrorist is likely to do? . . . There are terrorists who are highly organized, capable of using high technology and willing to kill thousands of people."[76]

Anthrax attacks in the United States in the fall of 2001, thought to be the work of an American bioterrorist, heightened fears that other microbes might be used as biological weapons. Anthrax broke out in several areas, including Florida, New Jersey, New York, and Washington, D.C. The anthrax, sent through the mail in the form of hardy spores, resulted in twenty-two illnesses and five deaths. Peter Jahrling, a scientist at America's principal biodefense laboratory, the United States Army Medical Research Institute of Infectious Diseases (USAMRIID), noted, "Anthrax does not spread as a contagious disease—you can't catch anthrax from someone who has it . . . but smallpox could spread through North America like wildfire." [77]

Preparing for a Smallpox Attack

Experts on biological warfare think smallpox would be a likely bioweapon because it is a stable microorganism, could be dispersed as an aerosol (spray), and is readily spread from person to person. A *New York Times* editorial published in June 2002 noted, "Should smallpox be delivered by aerosol in this country, the epidemic could spread much more rapidly than any outbreaks the public health system has previously encountered." [78] Although a smallpox spray would be the most efficient means of dispersing Variola, the virus could also be spread by contaminated objects, such as handkerchiefs, clothing, or towels. Richard Butler, the former head of the United Nations weapons-inspection teams in Iraq, observed, "Everyone wonders what kinds of delivery systems Iraq may have for biological weapons, but it seems to me that the best delivery system would be a suitcase left in the Washington subway." [79]

In the event of a surprise smallpox attack, the time between release of the virus and diagnosis of the first cases could be as long as two weeks or more, since the average incubation period for Variola is twelve to fourteen days. Because early detection and rapid response would help the government launch an effective defense, scientists are seeking a diagnostic test to identify Variola *earlier* in the illness. For this reason, scientists at the Centers for Disease Control are researching gene-based tests, which could detect smallpox even before the rash appears. These tests are not yet available, but scientists hope to develop them in the near future.

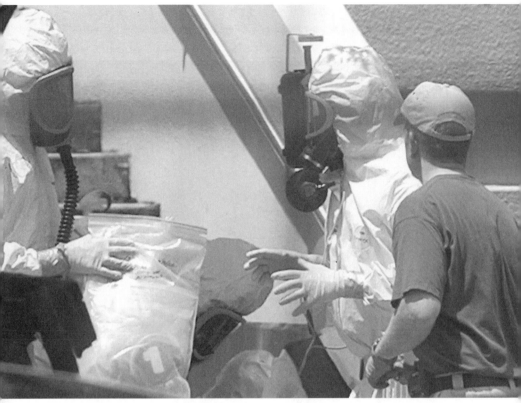

Workers wearing protective biohazard suits gather clues and infected debris from the former headquarters for the National Enquirer *after an anthrax attack in 2002.*

The Controversy over Vaccination

To get ready for a possible smallpox attack, the U.S. government is preparing a large stockpile of vaccine. This includes more than half a billion doses of "old" vaccine (which have been locked in storage facilities since 1972, when the United States ended routine vaccination) and several hundred million doses of "new" vaccine, now being produced by drug companies. Dr. Anthony Fauci, of the National Institute of Allergy and Infectious Diseases, observed, "In an emergency, we'd have enough to vaccinate everybody tomorrow."[80] The federal government has also called for cities and states to set up numerous clinics, which could open quickly during a smallpox emergency and—if necessary—vaccinate the entire population.

However, there is debate over whether or not the general population should receive smallpox vaccinations prior to an imminent attack. Some doctors believe widespread "peacetime" vaccination would be advantageous. Because the United States stopped routine vaccination in 1972, few Americans under the age of thirty have been vaccinated. Even individuals who were vaccinated years ago

Dr. Sharon Frey injects a woman with a diluted dose of smallpox vaccine. Some doctors encourage a return to routine vaccination to rebuild immunity to smallpox.

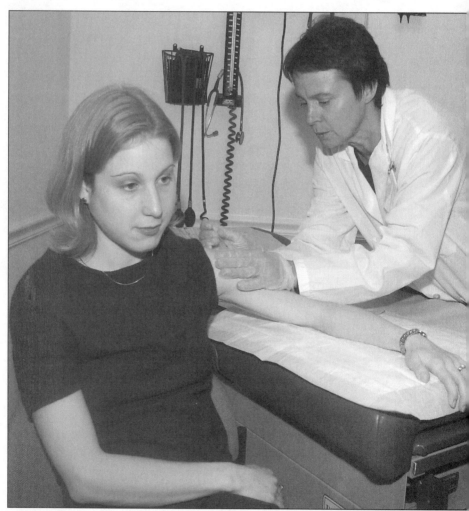

are now susceptible to the disease, since immunity wanes over time. Thus, residents of the United States and, in fact, the entire world are now susceptible to smallpox. Donald Millar, who participated in the smallpox eradication program decades ago, noted that mass vaccination of Americans would restore some of the population's lost immunity. Some doctors also think that people who develop vaccination side effects could be treated more easily during peacetime, when clinics are not overwhelmed.

Other physicians do not think mass peacetime vaccination is a good idea, since smallpox vaccinations can be dangerous. Complications occur in about one hundred of every 1 million people vaccinated, with a death rate of one per million. Vaccinia immune globulin (VIG) can be used to treat vaccination side effects. Nevertheless, Dr. O'Toole disapproves of large-scale vaccination. She notes, "This is a powerful vaccine, and some portion of the population can have serious, even fatal, reactions. If there were a clear threat of smallpox, the risk equation would change."[81]

The ideal solution—a vaccine without side effects—may soon be a reality. Scientists are beginning to test vaccines based on a weakened strain of vaccinia called modified vaccinia ankara (MVA). If MVA vaccines prove to be safe *and* effective, mass vaccination could again protect the world from smallpox.

Dark Winter: A Mock Smallpox Attack

The fear that enemies might attack the United States with biological weapons has been increasing since the early 1990s. Moreover, American authorities think rogue states such as Iraq, and possibly terrorist groups, may be producing smallpox weapons. To increase awareness of the type of threat posed by a smallpox attack, U.S. government officials participated in a war game called Dark Winter in June 2001.

The participants in the Dark Winter exercise gathered in a room, where they were presented with a set of fictional events. They then had to determine what their response would be if these incidents had actually occurred. Government officials and other people played the roles of president of the United States, national security adviser, director of the Central Intelligence Agency, secretary of defense, chairman of the Joint Chiefs of Staff, secretary of health and human services, director of the Federal Emergency Management Agency, director of the Federal Bureau of Investigation, governor of Oklahoma, correspondents for news organizations, and several others.

As the exercise began, the participants pretended that smallpox attacks had been launched in three shopping malls on December 1, 2002. It was determined that, using a total of only thirty grams (about one ounce) of smallpox virus, bioterrorists would have infected three thousand people in Oklahoma City, Philadelphia, and Atlanta. These victims would have constituted the "first wave" of smallpox cases.

In the game, it was assumed that the first signs of a smallpox attack would have come eight days later, when people with rashes would have shown up at emergency rooms and doctors' offices. By that time, the patients would have been contagious and spreading the virus to the "second wave" of victims. It was presumed that most doctors, being unfamiliar with smallpox, would not have immediately identified the illness. The delayed diagnosis would have allowed the disease to spread further.

Once government officials realized that a smallpox epidemic was occurring, they would have had to decide who would be vaccinated. For the game, it was assumed that only 12 million doses of vaccine were available. The participants pretended to choose the "ring vaccination plan." This would have restricted vaccination to those persons most likely to contract smallpox, including people who had come in contact with victims, health care workers, and public safety employees.

The participants then pretended that on December 15, 2002, two weeks after the attack, two thousand smallpox cases had been reported in fifteen states, with three hundred deaths. By then, the epidemic would also have spread to other countries, so a few cases would have appeared in Canada, Mexico, and Great Britain. By this time, there would have been only 1.25 million doses of vaccine left in the United States, and the public would have begun to panic.

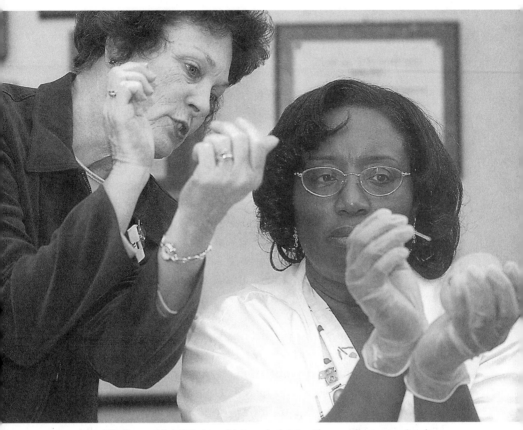

A public nurse (right) is taught to administer the smallpox vaccine by pricking an orange. Such training is designed to prepare health workers for the possibility of a bioterrorist attack.

Vaccine distribution would have varied from state to state, and people would have struggled to get to areas with larger stockpiles. Health care facilities would have been swamped. Several countries would have closed their borders to American trade and travel. Food supplies would have dwindled because of travel problems and closed stores.

In the game, it was assumed that U.S. drug companies would have been able to produce new vaccine at the rate of 6 million doses per month, with the first batch available after five weeks. It was also presumed that Russia would have provided 4 million doses of vaccine.

The players pretended that, on December 22, 2002, three weeks after the attack, sixteen thousand smallpox cases would have been reported in twenty-five states, with one thousand deaths. Smallpox would have spread to ten other countries. Vaccine supplies would have been gone, and new vaccine would not have been ready for a month. Residents of affected cities would have tried to flee. States would have restricted most travel, food shortages would have been increasing, and the nation's economy would have been suffering.

Canada and Mexico would have closed their borders to the United States. The public would have been demanding that smallpox victims and their contacts be quarantined, but locating all contacts would have become impossible. It was assumed that seventeen thousand additional smallpox cases would have appeared in the next twelve days, bringing the total number of second-wave victims to thirty thousand. Ten thousand of these people would have been expected to die.

In the game, the *worst-case* predictions were three hundred thousand third-wave victims, with one hundred thousand deaths, and 3 million fourth-wave cases, with 1 million deaths. It was assumed that the number of cases would have been lowered by large-scale vaccination programs and quarantine procedures.

The participants in the Dark Winter exercise assumed that American authorities would have been faced with daunting challenges and difficult questions, such as How would they stop the spread of smallpox with limited vaccine? Should patients and their contacts be quarantined in "smallpox facilities"? Should schools be closed? Should the government restrict travel? Should public events be suspended? What would be the best method of containing the disease while sustaining the economy and protecting civil liberties? What should the government do to care for the sick? Should military personnel be sent to assist in hospitals and clinics when they might be needed overseas? Should troops be sent to sensitive parts of the world? What should the president tell the people of the United States? Who are the bioterrorists? and so on. These issues led to intense debate among the game players.

Lessons Learned

Many lessons were learned from the Dark Winter exercise. First, it became clear that—at the time of the game—the United States was unprepared for the consequences of a bioterrorist attack. American authorities were unfamiliar with public health programs and un-acquainted with methods of caring for huge numbers of sick people. James Woolsey, the former director of central intelligence, said,

> We are used to thinking about health problems as naturally oc-curring problems outside the framework of a malicious actor [bioterrorist]. . . . If you're going against someone who is using a tool that you're not used to having him use [like] disease, and using it . . . quite rationally and craftily . . . [toward] an entirely unreasonable . . . end, we are in a world we haven't ever really been in before.[82]

Second, a deficiency of smallpox vaccine would have severely limited the ability of health care officials to control a smallpox epidemic. A vaccine shortage would also have led to conflict and flight among people desperate to get vaccinated. Governor Frank Keating of Oklahoma observed, "Who do you choose and who do you not choose to get vaccinated? . . . People are going to go where the vaccine is. And if they know that you're going to provide the vaccine . . . they'll stay to get vaccinated. I think they'll run if they think the vaccine is somewhere else."[83]

Third, the U.S. health care system at the time lacked the capacity to deal with mass casualties. In the Dark Winter scenario, hospital systems across the country would have been overwhelmed with patients. Insufficient health care resources, combined with a shortage of doctors and nurses, would have imposed an enormous burden on health care facilities.

Overall, Dark Winter demonstrated that an attack on the United States with bioweapons could cause massive casualties, a break-down of democratic processes, civil disorder, disruption of gov-ernment institutions, and a diminished ability to respond to military emergencies.

After studying the lessons of Dark Winter, U.S. administrators developed a strategy to protect civilian populations in the event of a smallpox attack. First, the United States would purchase and stockpile large quantities of vaccine. Second, American authorities would order the "prevaccination" of people most likely to be exposed. Tommy Thompson, secretary of health and human services, presented the White House with a plan for prevaccinating up to 10 million individuals, including health care employees, law enforcement officers, disease detectives, transportation workers, emer-

Tommy Thompson, secretary of health, advocated a prevaccination plan in which millions of people most likely to respond to a smallpox outbreak are vaccinated as a precautionary measure.

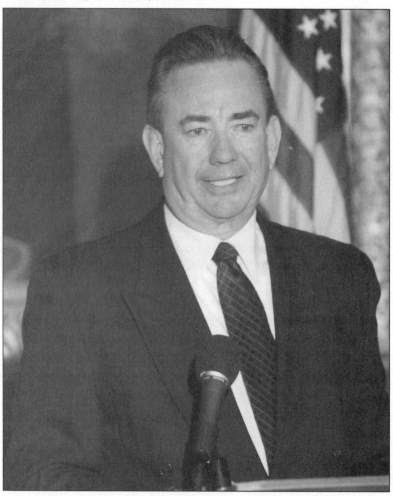

gency management staff, lab technicians, military personnel, and funeral home attendants. Many of these people would be "first responders," the first people to react in the event of a smallpox strike. Implementation of the prevaccination plan began in December 2002, when President George W. Bush ordered the immediate vaccination of about five hundred thousand soldiers and four hundred and fifty thousand emergency workers. The president was vaccinated also, declaring, "As commander-in-chief, I do not believe I can ask others to accept this risk unless I am willing to do the same. Therefore, I will receive the vaccine along with our military."[84] Starting in early 2003, millions of other civilians, including police, firefighters, and people participating in tests of unlicensed (trial) vaccines, would also be vaccinated. Moreover, the government planned to have licensed vaccines available to the general public by 2004 for anyone who wanted to be prevaccinated.

Plans were also made to train health care providers to recognize smallpox, and to set up numerous facilities to isolate and treat victims. Finally, it was decided that large amounts of VIG would be obtained to treat the possible side effects of vaccination.

Thus, in the event of a smallpox assault, health care workers would ideally be able to detect the disease quickly. Once smallpox was diagnosed, the victims would be isolated and their contacts would be vaccinated and monitored. Vaccination within four days of exposure would confer limited protection against infection and considerable protection against death. Simultaneous, rapid vaccination of the rest of the (previously unvaccinated) population would provide widespread immunity. With these plans in place, government officials believe that America would prevail against a smallpox attack.

Notes

Introduction: A Disease "Most Fearful to Behold"

1. Quoted in Jonathan B. Tucker, *Scourge: The Once and Future Threat of Smallpox*. New York: Atlantic Monthly Press, 2001, p. 11.
2. Quoted in Elizabeth A. Fenn, *Pox Americana: The Great Smallpox Epidemic of 1775–82*. New York: Hill & Wang, 2001, p. 18.
3. Quoted in James Cross Giblin, *When Plague Strikes: The Black Death, Smallpox, AIDS*. New York: HarperCollins, 1995, p. 63.

Chapter 1: What Is Smallpox?

4. Quoted in Donald R. Hopkins, *Princes and Peasants: Smallpox in History*. Chicago: University of Chicago Press, 1983, p. 234.
5. Richard Preston, "The Demon in the Freezer: How Smallpox, a Disease Officially Eradicated Twenty Years Ago, Became the Biggest Bioterrorist Threat We Now Face," *New Yorker*, July 12, 1999. http://cryptome.org.
6. Richard Preston, *The Demon in the Freezer: A True Story*. New York: Random House, 2002, p. 29.
7. Preston, "The Demon in the Freezer."
8. Preston, *The Demon in the Freezer*, p. 29.
9. Quoted in Preston, "The Demon in the Freezer."

Chapter 2: The Scourge and Its History

10. Quoted in Giblin, *When Plague Strikes*, p. 60.
11. Quoted in Hopkins, *Princes and Peasants*, p. 200.
12. Quoted in *American Life Histories: Manuscripts from the Federal Writers' Project, 1936–1940*. American Heritage Memory Projects, http://memory.loc.gov.
13. Quoted in Giblin, *When Plague Strikes*, p. 70.

14. Quoted in Giblin, *When Plague Strikes*, pp. 73–74.
15. Quoted in Giblin, *When Plague Strikes*, p. 75.
16. Quoted in Giblin, *When Plague Strikes*, pp. 75–76.
17. Quoted in Giblin, *When Plague Strikes*, p. 76.
18. Quoted in Fenn, *Pox Americana*, p. 176.
19. Quoted in Fenn, *Pox Americana*, p. 187.
20. Quoted in "Journal Entries," in *Migration of Disease: Smallpox.* www.geocities.com.
21. Quoted in Giblin, *When Plague Strikes*, p. 100.
22. Quoted in Hopkins, *Princes and Peasants*, pp. 272–73.

Chapter 3: Inoculation to Prevent Epidemics
23. Quoted in Tucker, *Scourge*, p. 3.
24. Quoted in Hopkins, *Princes and Peasants*, pp. 47–48.
25. Quoted in Giblin, *When Plague Strikes*, p. 81.
26. Quoted in Andrew Dickson White, "Theological Opposition to Inoculation, Vaccination, and the Use of Anaesthetics," in *A History of the Warfare of Science with Theology in Christendom*, 1898. www.santafe.edu.
27. Quoted in Fenn, *Pox Americana*, p. 32.
28. Quoted in Giblin, *When Plague Strikes*, p. 84.
29. Quoted in Fenn, *Pox Americana*, p. 41.
30. Quoted in Tucker, *Scourge*, p. 20.
31. Quoted in Tucker, *Scourge*, p. 20.
32. Quoted in Tucker, *Scourge*, p. 20.
33. Quoted in Tucker, *Scourge*, p. 20.
34. Quoted in Hopkins, *Princes and Peasants*, p. 258.
35. Quoted in Hopkins, *Princes and Peasants*, p. 258.
36. Quoted in Hopkins, *Princes and Peasants*, p. 261.
37. Quoted in Hopkins, *Princes and Peasants*, p. 262.
38. Quoted in Fenn, *Pox Americana*, p. 112.

Chapter 4: The Smallpox Vaccine Is Developed
39. Quoted in American College of Physicians/American Society of Internal Medicine Online, *Medicine in Quotations Online.* www.acponline.org.
40. Quoted in Giblin, *When Plague Strikes*, pp. 94–95.
41. Quoted in Giblin, *When Plague Strikes*, p. 95.

42. Quoted in *The Vaccination Experiments of Benjamin Waterhouse*, a catalog of the Benjamin Waterhouse exhibit at the Francis A. Countway Library of Medicine, Countway Library of Medicine, Rare Books and Special Collections, Harvard University. www.countway.med.harvard.edu.

43. Quoted in Paul Saunders, *Edward Jenner, the Cheltenham Years 1795–1823: Being a Chronicle of the Vaccination Campaign*, Hanover, NH: University Press of New England, 1982, p. 90.

44. Quoted in Saunders, *Edward Jenner*, p. 90.

45. Quoted in Saunders, *Edward Jenner*, p. 103.

46. Quoted in Alvin Powell, "The Beginning of the End of Smallpox: Medical School Professor Benjamin Waterhouse First to Test Vaccine in the U.S.," *Harvard University Gazette*, May 20, 1999. www.news.harvard.edu.

47. Quoted in *The Vaccination Experiments of Benjamin Waterhouse*.

48. Quoted in *The Vaccination Experiments of Benjamin Waterhouse*.

49. Quoted in Hopkins, *Princes and Peasants*, p. 265.

50. Quoted in Nicolau Barquet and Pere Domingo, "Smallpox: The Triumph over the Most Terrible Ministers of Death," *Annals of Internal Medicine*, October 15, 1997. www.acponline.org.

51. Quoted in Hopkins, *Princes and Peasants*, p. 271.

52. Quoted in Saunders, *Edward Jenner*, p. 193.

53. Quoted in Hopkins, *Princes and Peasants*, p. 87.

54. Quoted in S. Martin, "Anti-Vaccinationists Past and Present," *pkids Archives*, August 25, 2002. http://archive.mail-list.com.

55. Quoted in Hopkins, *Princes and Peasants*, p. 84.

56. Quoted in "How Was Vaccination Invented?" in *Immunisation: The Safest Way to Protect Your Child*. www.immunisation.org.uk.

57. Quoted in White, "Theological Opposition to Inoculation, Vaccination, and the Use of Anaesthetics."

58. Quoted in Giblin, *When Plague Strikes*, p. 97.

59. Quoted in Saunders, *Edward Jenner*, p. 112.

60. Quoted in Michael B.A. Oldstone, *Viruses, Plagues, and History*, Oxford, England: Oxford University Press, 1998, p. 40.

61. Quoted in Edward F. Dolan Jr., *Jenner and the Miracle of Vaccine*, New York: Dodd, Mead, 1960, pp. 40–41.

62. Quoted in Hopkins, *Princes and Peasants*, p. 82.

63. Quoted in Vaccine Website, "Smallpox Vaccination and Spread of Disease." www.whale.to/vaccine/small.html.

64. Quoted in Vaccine Website, "Smallpox Vaccination and Spread of Disease."

Chapter 5: Smallpox Is Eradicated

65. Quoted in Tucker, *Scourge*, pp. 44–45.

66. Quoted in Vaccine Website, "Smallpox Vaccination Quotes." www.whale.to/vaccine/smallpox_quotes.html.

67. Quoted in Tod Mohamed, "Exterminating an Age-Old Killer," (Ottawa) *Citizen's Weekly*, July 12, 1998. www.chrcrm.org.

68. Quoted in Mohamed, "Exterminating an Age-Old Killer."

69. Quoted in *People's Century*, "Interview with Zafar Husain, Smallpox Campaigner, India." www.pbs.org.

70. Quoted in Hans G. Andersson, "Interview with John Scott Porterfield, Smallpox Eradication Program Volunteer (1971)," *Biohazard News*, p. 1. www.biohazardnews.net/porterfield.

71. Quoted in Andersson, "Interview with John Scott Porterfield."

72. Quoted in Mohamed, "Exterminating an Age-Old Killer."

73. Quoted in Peter Thompson, "The Wisdom Interviews: Frank Fenner," *ABC Radio National*, September 1, 2002. www.abc.net.au.

Chapter 6: Smallpox as a Biological Weapon

74. Quoted in *Biohazard News*, "Smallpox as a Disease Agent," 2001. www.biohazardnews.net.

75. Quoted in Richard Preston, "Annals of Warfare: The Bioweaponeers," *New Yorker*, March 9, 1998. http://cryptome.org.

76. Quoted in BBC Online, "Hot Topics: Questions and Answers About the Smallpox Threat," April 15, 2002. www.bbc.co.uk.

77. Quoted in Preston, *The Demon in the Freezer*, p. 29.

78. *New York Times*, "How to Prepare for a Smallpox Attack," June 23, 2002. www.nytimes.com.

79. Quoted in Preston, "Annals of Warfare."

80. Quoted in Geoffrey Cowley, "The Plan to Fight Smallpox," *Newsweek*, October 14, 2002, pp. 48–49.

81. Quoted in BBC Online, "Questions and Answers About the Smallpox Threat."

82. Quoted in Michael Mair O'Toole and Thomas V. Inglesby, "Shining Light on 'Dark Winter,'" *Clinical Infectious Diseases*, February 19, 2002. www.journals.uchicago.edu/CID.

83. Quoted in O'Toole and Inglesby, "Shining Light on 'Dark Winter.'"

84. Quoted in Associated Press, "President Vaccinated Against Smallpox," *Washington Times*, December 22, 2002. www.wash times.com.

Glossary

antibiotic: A medicine that can destroy harmful bacteria in the body or limit their growth; used to treat bacterial infections.

antibodies: Protein molecules produced by the body to kill germs, fight disease, and eliminate foreign substances.

cidofovir: A drug that interferes with DNA replication that may help prevent smallpox if given within a day or two of exposure.

complications: Additional medical problems caused by an illness or a vaccination.

Dark Winter: A war game conducted by American officials in June 2001 to increase awareness of the type of threat posed by a surprise smallpox attack on the United States.

DNA (deoxyribonucleic acid): A chemical substance that usually makes up chromosomes; composes the genetic material of some viruses.

enzyme: A chemical substance produced by living cells that regulates the speed of body processes.

immune system: The body system that defends the body against infection, disease, and foreign substances.

inoculation: A procedure in which a person is deliberately infected with a mild form of smallpox to protect the individual from more deadly forms of the disease.

pustule: A vesicle (blister) on the skin that contains pus.

RNA (ribonucleic acid): A chemical substance that is usually associated with the control of cellular chemical activities; composes the genetic material of some viruses.

vaccine: A substance that, when introduced into the body, induces immunity to a disease; usually contains part of, or a harmless form of, the virus or bacteria that causes the disease.

Variola: Scientific name for the smallpox virus; it comes in two types, Variola major (which causes more serious forms of smallpox) and Variola minor (which causes milder forms of smallpox).

VIG (vaccinia immune globulin): A medicine used to treat the side effects of smallpox vaccinations.

virus: An extremely small life-form that can reproduce only inside living cells, using the cells' machinery; viruses cause diseases in humans, animals, and plants.

Organizations to Contact

Armed Forces Institute of Pathology (AFIP)
6825 16th St. NW
Washington, DC 20306-6000
(202) 782-2100
www.afip.org
The AFIP is an agency of the Department of Defense specializing in pathology consultation, education, and research. It provides extensive information about infectious diseases.

Centers for Disease Control and Prevention (CDC)
1600 Clifton Rd.
Atlanta, GA 30333
(404) 639-3311
www.cdc.gov
The CDC is the lead federal agency for protecting the health and safety of people. It provides extensive information about public health and contagious diseases.

Pan American Health Organization
Pan American Sanitary Bureau
Regional Office of the World Health Organization
525 Twenty-third St. NW
Washington, DC 20037
(202) 974-3000
www.paho.org
The Pan American Health Organization is an international public health agency that provides extensive information about public health and contagious diseases.

For Further Reading

Arthur Diamond, *Smallpox and the American Indian*. San Diego: Lucent Books, 1991. A history of the smallpox epidemics that decimated Native Americans in the 1800s.

Margaret O. Hyde and Elizabeth H. Forsyth, *Vaccinations: From Smallpox to Cancer*. New York: Franklin Watts, 2000. A description of several illnesses with details about how vaccines prepare the immune system to fight disease.

A.J. Harding Rains, *Pioneers of Science and Discovery: Edward Jenner and Vaccination*. East Sussex, England: Wayland, 1980. A biography of Edward Jenner focusing on his efforts to promote smallpox vaccination.

Tom Ridgway, *Epidemics, Deadly Diseases Throughout History: Smallpox*. New York: Rosen, 2001. An account of the cause, history, and eradication of smallpox.

Works Consulted

Books

George Catlin, *North American Indians.* New York: Viking Penguin, 1996. Descriptions and drawings of Native Americans who lived in the American West during the 1830s.

Edward F. Dolan Jr., *Jenner and the Miracle of Vaccine.* New York: Dodd, Mead, 1960. A biography of Edward Jenner, written in the style of a novel.

Elizabeth A. Fenn, *Pox Americana: The Great Smallpox Epidemic of 1775–82.* New York: Hill & Wang, 2001. A detailed study of smallpox epidemics during the American Revolution, including their effect on the war.

Bill Frist, *When Every Moment Counts: What You Need to Know About Bioterrorism from the Senate's Only Doctor.* Lantham, MD: Rowan & Littlefield, 2002. A discussion of biological weapons and the steps people can take to protect themselves against a biological attack.

James Cross Giblin, *When Plague Strikes: The Black Death, Smallpox, AIDS.* New York: HarperCollins, 1995. A discussion of the black death, smallpox, and AIDS and the devastation they caused.

Donald R. Hopkins, *Princes and Peasants: Smallpox in History.* Chicago: University of Chicago Press, 1983. An extensive study of the impact of smallpox on the history of the world.

Geoffrey Marks and William K. Beatty, *Epidemics.* New York: Charles Scribner's Sons, 1976. A discussion of the epidemics that have plagued humankind from ancient to recent times.

Michael B.A. Oldstone, *Viruses, Plagues, and History.* Oxford, England: Oxford University Press, 1998. An account of the ways in which deadly viruses have affected civilizations through time.

Richard Preston, *The Demon in the Freezer: A True Story.* New York: Random House, 2002. An extensive discussion of the use of smallpox as a biological weapon.

Ed Regis, *Virus Ground Zero: Stalking the Killer Viruses with the Centers for Disease Control.* New York: Pocket Books, 1996. A behind-the-scenes description of the procedures used by the Centers for Disease Control to track killer viruses.

Paul Saunders, *Edward Jenner, the Cheltenham Years 1795–1823: Being a Chronicle of the Vaccination Campaign.* Hanover, NH: University Press of New England, 1982. A biography that focuses on Edward Jenner's campaign to vaccinate people against smallpox in the late 1700s and 1800s.

Jonathan B. Tucker, *Scourge: The Once and Future Threat of Smallpox.* New York: Atlantic Monthly Press, 2001. A portrayal of the battles waged by human populations against smallpox throughout history.

Periodicals

Geoffrey Cowley, "The Plan to Fight Smallpox," *Newsweek,* October 14, 2002.

Anita Manning, "U.S. Ramps Up Bioterror Plan: Mass Vaccination in Case of Smallpox," *USA Today,* September 24, 2002.

Internet Sources

American College of Physicians/American Society of Internal Medicine Online, *Medicine in Quotations Online.* www.acponline.org.

American Heritage Memory Projects, *American Life Histories: Manuscripts from the Federal Writers' Project, 1936–1940.* http://memory.loc.gov.

Hans G. Andersson, "Interview with John Scott Porterfield, Smallpox Eradication Program Volunteer (1991)," *Biohazard News.* www.biohazardnews.net.

Associated Press, "President Vaccinated Against Smallpox," *Washington Times,* December 22, 2002. www.washtimes.com.

Nicolau Barquet and Pere Domingo, "Smallpox: The Triumph over the Most Terrible Ministers of Death," *Annals of Internal Medicine,* October 15, 1997. www.acponline.org.

BBC Online, "Hot Topics: Questions and Answers About the Smallpox Threat," April 15, 2002. www.bbc.co.uk.

Biohazard News, "Smallpox as a Disease Agent," 2001. www.biohazard news.net.

Keith Bradsher, "The Treatment: U.S. Begins Search for Medicine Used to Treat Adverse Reactions to Smallpox Vaccine," *New York Times,* October 22, 2001. www.homeopathicservices.com.

Anthony Browne, "UN's Smallpox Terror Alert," *Observer,* October 21, 2001. www.observer.co.uk.

Frank Buckley and Elizabeth Cohen, "Bush Orders Smallpox Vaccine for Military, Himself," CNN, December 17, 2002. http://asia.cnn.com.

Garance Franke-Ruta, "George Washington's Bioterrorism Strategy: How We Handled It Last Time," *Washington Monthly Online,* December 2001. www.washingtonmonthly.com.

D.A. Henderson et al., "Smallpox as a Biological Weapon," *Medical and Public Health Management,* June 9, 1999. http://jama.ama-assn.org.

"How Was Vaccination Invented?" in *Immunisation: The Safest Way to Protect Your Child.* www.immunisation.org.uk.

"Journal Entries," in *Migration of Disease: Smallpox.* www.geo cities.com.

Tom A. Kerns, *Jenner on Trial: The Ethics of Vaccine Research in the Age of Smallpox and the Age of AIDS,* University Press of America, 1997. (http://students.washington.edu.) An online book with chapters about smallpox, AIDS, and Edward Jenner's development of smallpox vaccine.

S. Martin, "Anti-Vaccinationists Past and Present," *pkids Archives,* August 25, 2002. http://archives.mail-list.com.

Tod Mohamed, "Exterminating an Age-Old Killer," (Ottawa) *Citizen's Weekly,* July 12, 1998. www.chrcrm.org.

Lauran Neergaard, "Scientists Work on Smallpox Medicines," *Washington Post,* June 2, 2002. www.amprogress.org.

New York Times, "How to Prepare for a Smallpox Attack," June 23, 2002. www.nytimes.com.

Michael Mair O'Toole and Thomas V. Inglesby, "Shining Light on 'Dark Winter,'" *Clinical Infectious Diseases*, February 19, 2002. www.journals.uchicago.edu/CID.

People's Century, "Interview with Zafar Husain, Smallpox Campaigner, India." www.pbs.org.

Alvin Powell, "The Beginning of the End of Smallpox: Medical School Professor Benjamin Waterhouse First to Test Vaccine in the U.S.," *Harvard University Gazette*, May 20, 1999. www.news.harvard.edu.

Richard Preston, "Annals of Warfare: The Bioweaponeers," *New Yorker*, March 9, 1998. http://cryptome.org.

———, "The Demon in the Freezer: How Smallpox, a Disease Officially Eradicated Twenty Years Ago, Became the Biggest Bioterrorist Threat We Now Face," *New Yorker*, July 12, 1999. http://cryptome.org.

Rafael E. Tarrago, "The Balmis-Salvany Smallpox Expedition: The First Public Health Vaccination Campaign in South America," *Perspectives in Health*, vol. 6, no. 1, 2001. www.paho.org.

Peter Thompson, "The Wisdom Interviews: Frank Fenner," *ABC Radio National*, September 1, 2002. www.abc.net.au.

Vaccination News, "The Vaccination Experiments of Benajamin Waterhouse: A Catalogue of the Benjamin Waterhouse Exhibit at the Francis A. Countway Library of Medicine," 2000. www.vaccinationnews.com.

Vaccine Website, "Smallpox Vaccination and Spread of Disease." www.whale.to/vaccine/small.html.

———, "Smallpox Vaccination Quotes." www.whale.to/vaccine/smallpox_quotes.html.

Andrew Dickson White, "Theological Opposition to Inoculation, Vaccination, and the Use of Anaesthetics," in *A History of the Warfare of Science with Theology in Christendom*, 1898. www.santafe.edu.

Websites

All the Virology on the WWW (www.virology.net). Contains extensive information about viruses.

Biohazard News (www.biohazardnews.net). A civilian initiative addressing the threat of bioterrorism; contains many articles and interviews related to bioterrorism.

Centers for Strategic and International Studies (www.csis.org). Contains information about current and emerging global issues, including medical and health concerns.

Countway Library of Medicine, Rare Books and Special Collections (www.countway.med.harvard.edu/rarebooks/waterhouse). Catalogs an exhibit of Benjamin Waterhouse's vaccination experiments.

Cowpox (http://duke.usask.ca/~misra/virology/stud2002/edo web/main.html). Contains discussions of various topics related to the cowpox virus.

Division of Medical Microbiology, University of Capetown (http://web.uct.ac.za/depts/mmi). Contains discussions of various topics related to health care and the prevention of infectious diseases.

History Television: National Geographic Channel (www.history television.ca/chiefs). This website explores the lives and times of Native American leaders and discusses Native American smallpox epidemics.

Merck Manual of Diagnosis and Therapy (www.merck.com/pubs/ mmanual). Contains discussions of various topics related to medicine and health.

Migration of Disease: Smallpox (www.geocities.com/Athens/ Oracle/8492/index.html). Contains discussions of various topics related to smallpox, including Native American epidemics, vaccination, and general information about the disease.

MJA: The Medical Journal of Australia (www.mja.com.au). Contains articles about a large variety of medical topics.

On-Line Medical Dictionary, Department of Medical Oncology, University of Newcastle upon Tyne (http://cancerweb.ncl.ac.uk/omd). Dictionary of medical terms.

Poxviridae (www.stanford.edu/group/virus/pox/2000/index. html). Contains extensive information about poxviruses.

Radio National: The Health Report (www.abc.net.av/rn/talks/ 8.30/helthrpt). Contains numerous stories, interviews, and discussions related to public health topics.

UCLA Department of Epidemiology: School of Public Health (www.ph.vela.edu/epi). Contains information about epidemic diseases.

Vaccination News (www.vaccinationnews.com). Contains information and discussions about all sides of the vaccination controversy.

Vaccine Website (www.whale.to/vaccines.html). Contains extensive information about vaccine and vaccinations.

Index

Africa
  inoculations in, 35
  smallpox gods worshiped in,
     25
alastrim. *See* mild smallpox
Algonquian, 31
Alibek, Ken, 76
Amelia (Princess Caroline's
  daughter), 38
American Fur Company, 33
American Revolution, 42–46
Amherst, Jeffrey, 41–42
Andes Mountains, 29
anthrax, 10, 74, 78
antibiotics, 20, 36
Anti-Vaccination Society, 59
Arikara, 33
Arnold, Benedict, 45
arthritis, 18
Assiniboin, 33–34
Atahualpa, 29–30
Attila, 25
Aum Shinrikyo cult, 76
Australia, 75
Austria, 64
avipoxviruses, 12
Aztec, 28–29

bacterial infection, 16
Baillie, Matthew, 60
Balmis, Francis Xavier de, 57–58
Bangladesh, 70

Banister, Charles, 26
Baron, John, 53
Bavaria, 60
Bedson, Henry, 9
Berlin, 63
bifurcated needles, 68
bioterrorism
  anthrax attacks in United
     States, 10, 74, 78
  bioterrorists' access to Variola
     virus, 76–78
  destruction of Variola virus
     samples postponed, 72–73
  against Native Americans,
     41–42
  preparation for attacks from
     smallpox, 78–87
Birch, John, 59–60
Blackfoot, 33–34
bleeding, 25
blindness, 18
blood poisoning, 16
Bohemia, 60
Bombay, 65
Boston
  inoculations against smallpox
     in, 39–40
  opposition to smallpox
     vaccinations in, 59
  smallpox epidemics in, 32,
     42–44
Bouquet, Henry, 41–42

Boylston, Thomas, 39
Boylston, Zabdiel, 39–40
Bradford, William, 8
Brazil
    description of suffering from
        smallpox in, 8
    spread of smallpox in, 30
bronchitis, 17
Bush, George W., 87
Butler, Richard, 78

Canada
    Indians of, show
        appreciation to Jenner, 60
    outbreak of smallpox in, 32
    smallpox vaccinations in, 60,
        75
Capac, Huayna, 29
capripoxviruses, 12
Caroline (princess of Wales), 38
Caroline (Princess Caroline's
    daughter), 38
Carter, Samuel, 54
Catlin, George, 34, 56
CDC. *See* Centers for Disease
    Control
Centers for Disease Control
    (CDC)
    challenges in finding
        smallpox outbreaks by,
        68–70
    on dangers of smallpox as
        biological weapon, 74
    develops new vaccination
        methods, 68
    keeps Variola virus samples,
        72
    leads worldwide smallpox
        eradication campaign, 65
    smallpox research conducted
        by, 21, 78
Central America
    eradication of smallpox in, 64

spread of smallpox in, 27–30
Chardon, F.A., 34
Charles IV (king of Spain), 57
Charleston, South Carolina, 40
Chickasaw, 34
chicken pox, 19
Chiefs of Five Nations, 60
China
    inoculations against
        smallpox in, 35–36
    worship of smallpox goddess
        in, 23–24
Chisolm, Brock, 65
Choctaw, 34
cidofovir, 20
Cline, Henry, 58
College of Physicians, 38
Collier, Leslie, 67
Columbus, Christopher, 27
Comanche, 34
conjunctivitis, 18
Connecticut, 45
Constantinople, 36–37
contamination, 62
Continental Army, 42
Cortés, Hernando, 28–29
Costa, Italo, 71
cottonpox, 15
cowpox, 49–53, 67–68
    matter, 57–58, 61–62
    true, 53
Crow, 34
Cuba, 64
Cuban itch, 15
Cuzco, 29

"Dangerous and Sinful Practice
    of Inoculation, The"
    (sermon), 38
Dark Winter, 81–87
Denmark, 60
Dominican Republic. *See*
    Hispaniola

dung tea, 26

Ecuyer, Simeon, 42
eczema vaccinatum, 63
encephalitis, 17

Fauci, Anthony, 79
Fenner, Frank, 72
Flag, Kesiah, 54
Florida, 78
Foege, William, 71
Fort Clark, 33–34
Fort McKenzie, 34
Fort Union, 34
France
    patron saint of smallpox in, 25
    smallpox vaccinations in, 57
Franco-Prussian War, 63
Franklin, Benjamin, 41
French and Indian War, 41–42

Gantt, Edward, 56
generalized vaccinia, 63
George (prince of Wales), 38
Global Commission for the
    Certification of Smallpox
    Eradication, 72
Gloucestershire, 48, 50, 53
Great Britain
    eradication of smallpox in, 64
    inoculations in, 35–38
    smallpox vaccination
        program in, 60
Gregory of Tours, 8
Gros Ventres (tribe), 33–34

Haiti. *See* Hispaniola
Hemming, John, 30
hemorrhagic smallpox, 14, 20
Henderson, Donald Ainslie, 65,
    67
Herrlich, Albert, 65
Hidatsa, 33

Hispaniola, 27–30
History of England (Macaulay), 35
House of Commons, 60
Huáscar, 29
Hudson's Bay Company, 32
Hudson House trading post, 32
Huns, 25
Hunter, John, 49
Husain, Zafar, 70

immunity, 62
Inca, 28–30
India
    inoculations against smallpox
        in, 35–36
    outbreaks of smallpox in, 65
    virus hunters in, 70
    worship of smallpox goddess
        in, 22–23
inflammation, 16–18
inoculations
    of American colonists, 39–41
    during the American
        Revolution, 42–46
    in Great Britain, 35–38
    in Middle East, 35
    replaced by vaccinations,
        58–60
    in Russia, 35–36
    see also specific names of states
*Inquiry into the Causes and Effects
    of the Variolae Vaccinae, a
    Disease Discovered in Some of
    the Western Counties of
    England, Particularly
    Gloucestershire, and Known by
    the Name of Cowpox, An*
    (Edward Jenner), 51–52
Institute of Virus Preparations,
    72
iritis, 18
Iroquois, 32
Israel, 75

Italy, 62

Jahrling, Peter, 78
Japan, 24–25
Jefferson, Thomas, 55–56, 60
Jenner, Edward
    advocates vaccinations
        against smallpox, 51–52
    develops smallpox vaccine, 8,
        50–51
    early career of, 48–50
    receives recognition for
        vaccine, 60–61
    on Royal Smallpox
        Expedition, 58
Jenner, Robert, 50
Jenner, Stephen, 48
Jesuits, 30

Keating, Frank, 85
keratitis, 18
Kiowa, 34

leporipoxviruses, 12
Little Turtle, 56
Ludlow, Daniel, 49

Maalin, Ali Maow, 9, 71–72
Macaulay, Thomas Babington, 35
macules, 15–16
Madison, James, 60
Maitland, Charles, 37–38
malignant smallpox, 14, 20
Malthus, Thomas Robert, 59
Mandan, 33–34
Manila scab, 15
Marblehead, Massachusetts, 55
Maryland, 45
Massachusetts
    inoculations against
        smallpox in, 39–40
    smallpox epidemics in,
        31–32, 42–44, 55

Massey, Edward, 38
Mather, Increase, 31–32, 39
measles, 18, 26
Merca, 71
Mexico, 27–30
Mexico City, 32
Middle East, 35
mild smallpox, 15, 50
milkers' nodules, 49
Millar, Donald, 81
Mississippi River, 32
Missouri River, 32, 34
modified vaccinia ankara
    (MVA), 81
Mohamed, Tod, 71
monkeypox, 12, 22
Montagu, Edward, 37–38
Montagu, Mary (Mary
    Wortley's daughter), 37–38
Montagu, Mary Wortley, 36–38
Montezuma, 28–29
Montgomery, Richard, 45
Moravians, 47
Mutwa, Credo, 69–70
MVA. *See* modified vaccinia
    ankara

Napoleon, 57, 61
Narváez, Pánfilo de, 29
Native Americans
    Bradford describes suffering
        of, from smallpox, 8
    refuse to participate in
        smallpox vaccination
        program, 55
    spread of smallpox among,
        31–34
Nelmes, Sarah, 50
Newgate Prison, 38
New Jersey
    anthrax attacks in, 78
    inoculations against
        smallpox in, 45

New Orleans, 32
New York (state)
    anthrax attacks in, 78
    inoculations against smallpox
        in, 45
    smallpox outbreaks in, 32
New York City
    inoculations against smallpox
        in, 40
    outbreaks of smallpox in, 64
New York Times (newspaper), 78
Niang-Niang, T'ou-Shen, 23–24
Nicaise, Saint, 25
North Carolina, 47
North Church, 39
North Dakota, 33–34
North Saskatchewan River, 32
Norway, 60

Obaluaye, 25
Oman, Mitchell, 32
Omolu, 25
Onesimus, 39
Oregon Trail, 56
orthopoxviruses, 12
Osage (tribe), 34
Oshimoa, 25
osteomyelitis, 18
Osterholm, Michael, 75
O'Toole, Tara, 77, 81
Ottawa (tribe), 41–42

papules, 16
Parker, Janet, 9
Pawnee, 34
Pearson, George, 53
ped-o-jets, 68
Pennsylvania, 45
Pennsylvania Gazette
    (newspaper), 41
Peru, 29
pesthouses, 35
Philadelphia, 40–41
Philippines, 64

Phipps, James, 50
Pizarro, Francisco, 30
Plains Indians, 32–33
Plymouth Colony, 31–32
pneumonia, 17
pockmarks, 16
Pontiac (tribe), 41
Porterfield, John Scott, 70
postvaccinal encephalitis, 63
poxviruses, 12
Preston, Richard, 15–16, 19–20
progressive vaccinia, 63
*Prospect of Exterminating the
    Small Pox, A* (Benjamin
    Waterhouse), 54
Puerto Rico
    eradication of smallpox in, 64
    vaccination board in, 57–58
pustules, 16, 18, 36

al-Qaeda, 76
quarantine, 26, 35
Quebec, smallpox epidemics in,
    42, 45
Quetzalcoatl, 28–30

Ramses V, 22
rashes, 15–16
Reims, 25
Revolutionary War. *See*
    American Revolution
Royal Smallpox Expedition,
    57–58
Royal Society, 38
Russia
    deaths from smallpox in, 63
    inoculations against smallpox
        in, 35–36
    smallpox vaccination
        program in, 60

Sacco, Louis, 54
Sagbata, 25

Salem, North Carolina, 47
scars, 16
septicemia, 16
Shapona, 25
Sioux (tribe), 33–34
Sitala, 22–23
slaves, 27–29, 39
Sloane, Hans, 38
smallpox
  as biological weapon
    dangers of, 74–75
    see also bioterrorism
  complications from, 16–18
  diagnosis of, 18–20
  eradication of
    last case before, 71–72
    new vaccines developed
      for, 66–67
    role of virus hunters in,
      68–70
    surveillance and
      containment strategies
      for, 70–71
    worldwide campaign
      launched for, 64–66
  origin and spread of, 22
  prevention of
    through inoculations,
      35–41, 45–46
    through religious rituals,
      22–25
  spread of
    in Central and South
      America, 27–30
    death tolls from, 26–27
    in Hispaniola, 27–30
    among North American
      Indians, 31–34
    through trading posts,
      32–34
  symptoms of, 15–16
  treatment of
    antiviral medications for,

20–21
  folk remedies as, 25–26
  vaccine developed for, 8,
    50–51, 66–67
  types of, 14–15
  see also Variola virus
smallpox ships, 35
Snell, Powell, 53
Society for the Inoculation of
  the Poor, 41
Somalia, 71
South Africa, virus hunters in,
  69–70
South America, 27–30
Soviet Union
  eradication of smallpox in,
    64
  smallpox vaccinations in, 75
  Variola virus samples in, 72
Spain, 57–58
St. George's Hospital, 49
St. Pacras Smallpox Hospital,
  53
Sweden
  eradication of smallpox in, 64
  smallpox program in, 60
Switzerland, 63
syphilis, 8, 62

Tametomo, Chinzei Hachiro,
  24–25
Tebb, William, 62
Tenochtitlán, 29
Thompson, Tommy, 86–87
Thursfield, Hugh, 46
toxemia, 16
trading posts, 32–34
Trent, William, 42
Turkey, 35–36

United States
  bioterrorism in
    anthrax attacks, 10, 74, 78

against Native Americans, 41–42
eradication of smallpox in, 64
inoculations of colonists in, 39–41
smallpox vaccinations in, 54, 60, 75, 79–81
stages mock smallpox attack in, 81–87
Variola virus samples in, 72
University of Birmingham, 9

vaccination board, 57–58
vaccinations
  advocated by Edward Jenner, 51–52
  current controversies over, 79–81
  developed against smallpox, 8, 50–51, 66–67
  inoculations replaced by, 58–60
  of military personnel, 75
  problems with, 61–63
  by Royal Smallpox Expedition, 57–58
  spread to United States, 54
  supported by Jefferson, 55–56
vaccinia, 67–68
vaccinia immune globulin (VIG), 81, 87
Variola virus
  bioterrorists' access to, 76–78
  description of, 11–13
  destruction of samples of, postponed, 72–73
  escapes from a laboratory, 9
  identification of, 20

inoculations as protection from, 36
strains of, 14–15, 20
see also smallpox
variolation. *See* inoculations
vesicles, 16
VIG. *See* vaccinia immune globulin
Virginia, 45
viruses, 11–13
virus hunters, 68–70

Wagstaffe, William, 38
Ward, Nicholas, 20
War of Independence. *See* American Revolution
Washington, D.C., 78
Washington, George, 42–45
Waterhouse, Benjamin (doctor), 54–55
Waterhouse, Benjamin (son of Dr. Waterhouse), 54
Waterhouse, Daniel, 54
Waterhouse, Elizabeth, 54
Waterhouse, Mary, 54
West Indian smallpox, 15
whitepox, 15
WHO. *See* World Health Organization
Wickett, John, 70
Woodville, William, 53
Woolsey, James, 85
World Health Assembly, 65
World Health Organization (WHO), 64–65, 72–73, 75

York Factory trading post, 32
Yoruba, 25

Zhadnov, Viktor M., 65

Picture Credits

About the Author

Barbara Saffer, a former college instructor, has Ph.D. degrees in biology and geology. She writes fiction and nonfiction for children and has published books about science, geography, exploration, famous people, and historical events. She lives in Birmingham, Alabama, with her family.